The Ultimate Atkins Weight Loss Guide and Diet Recipes

Top Atkins Diet Recipes for Beginners

By Flat Belly Queens

Published in Great Britain by:

Flat Belly Queens
345 Old Street
London
EC1V 9LE

© Copyright 2016 – Flatbelly Queens

ISBN-13: {978-1533216373}
ISBN-10: {1533216371}

Table of Contents

Introduction:

The modern era is regarded as the climax of progress and development. Every single item of utility presented for our use is now dependent upon technology. From a simple mobile phone to a sophisticated space shuttle, everything around us is technology oriented. We do not have to put ourselves into the pain of manual labor; the result is obvious in the shape of extreme ease in our lives.

The addition of technology is not only limited to physical needs. Even the intake of this modern prepared with the utmost utility of technology. But to this height, there is a downside. The excessive utility in the form of technology has ruined the inclination towards physical activity. Similarly, the advent of processed and artificial food has made us far away from natural eatables. Fresh fruits and vegetables are stories of the past. The result of this extreme sophistication is evident in the form of obesity.

Every segment and every gender of the population are now worried aboutweight loss. Even young people are complaining of excessive weight gain. In this case, there is a need for some miraculous diet plan which can save us all, without compromising the quality of life. Here is the first step towards that miracle. It is none other than Atkins Diet. It is a complete package for sustaining a vigorous life with ideal weight condition, unlike another diet plan Atkins diet will save you from starvation but results will be more than obvious. Let's start the venture.

Chapter 1:

HOW DOES ATKINS WORK

Why consider "diet"

In today's world of rapid advancements put forward by technology and innovation, the human life has begun to transform a lot. There has been a rapid change in life patterns and working routines. The concept of economic pressures and financial challenges has led everyone to struggle even more for individual betterment. Although human race is moving towards an overall progress and accelerated rate of development, yet there are a number of hidden or overlooked consequences. These include the inability to look for plans. All these result in enhanced number of body ailments and an increased rate of obesity. Even if obesity is not there, the overall body composition of modern man is not enough for pertaining optimum levels of energy. It has become a global dilemma which needs to be addressed. Globally there is an intense need to revisit out eating patterns and tendencies to indulge in unhealthy diet plans.

A need for revolutionary diet approach

Based upon the above argument, there is a need for following some revolutionary approach of diet which can:

- ➤ Enable us to shed weight, without losing calories.
- ➤ Make us feel better from with and displays its significance in the form of healthy looks
- ➤ Facilitate a natural vitality in the body you.
- ➤ Enable a permanent solution against extra pounds so that weight shedding is not temporary.
- ➤ Serve the human body requirements with healthy diet recipes, without a need for compromising the delight of our tastebuds.

So in order to fulfill these requirements, the

additional benefits.

Atkins diet! Revolutionary approach

The Atkins nutritional approach or diet is known to be a low-carbohydrate approach. The reason for calling it a revolutionary approach is its ability to make the human body healthier after following the approach in true meanings. In contrast to other diet plans, which make the body feel lethargic and tired, Atkins diet reenergizes the body and enhances the inner vigor of the body.

The crown of introducing this revolution for human life is labeled to Robert Atkinsandhen the diet got the name, Atkins.

Atkins, while studying and searching about his weight issues, came to this method of weight loss. Overwhelmed with the consequences on weight issues and additional benefits, he started writing about it in series of different books so that general public can get the advantage of this fabulous method. He used the study to resolve his own overweight condition. The original method was introduced in 1972 and then various updated versions came on following the way. Various other nutritional experts and researchers then contributed in this innovative method of weight loss.

Chapter 2:

Benefits of Atkins diet

If you are new to learn this mode of diet, you must be curious about learning the exceptional benefits which one can ensure after following this approach. This comparison is natural as one can decide after comparing the true potentials of Atkins Diet plan with other traditional methods applied for weight loss.

The principles governing Atkins diet approach are all extended in a way which keeps in mind the natural biological and physiological needs of human body. Being naturally inclined, Atkins diet does not induces any artificial or imposed results on the body so whatever is achieved, it is helpful for overall betterment

1. Weight loss is focus but optimum weight is the pivotal point

This diet plan will make sure that the follower loses weight. Using this approach of nutritional intake losing weight is not an issue. There is no gender discrimination in the case of results, both women and men undergo thorough same body tuning. So the weight losing results will be the same in shedding weight and losing inches. There can be some unusual cases as well who possess the natural metabolic resistance against pound shedding. But Atkins diet has special considerations for these issues.

Atkins diet works on optimizing the body weight. It means that for every individual ideal body weight will vary so there can be no hard and fast rule for ideal weight. Maintaining the optimum body weight is not related to body shape only but it is also necessary for keeping the body away from various other body ailments and health issues. So Atkins does not believe on cosmetic benefits of weight loss which only intend to make the body look attractive. Rather Atkins believes on attainment of an overall healthy stage for the body.

2. Maintenance of optimum weight condition

One of the most distinguishing features of Atkins diet is to enable the body to maintain the ideal weight condition. This is the best result which ant nutritional approach can extend and Atkins in known for it. You can see many of the dieting plans and work out sessions which push the person to lose weight within two to three months. But whenever the person leaves the whole plan even for a few days, the whole weight is gained back. It is the point at where people feel disappointed and hopeless. But the root cause of weight coming back is the low fat approach to traditional diet plans. In these diet plans people are redistricted from fat consumption, which is possible only for a few days. As a result whenever fat consumption is restored, the body weight comes to the original point.

Traditional diet plans are based on the principle of starvation. Hunger is not easy to control. It requires stamina and a strong commitment. Therefore Atkins diet plan negates this unnatural way of losing weight and keeping the body hungry. Atkins diet strategy is to include enough of protein and fat in one's meals so that hunger can not disturb the body. The Atkins diet approach is moderate and negates extremism. The moderate approach ensures permanent results.

3. Achievement of health and vitality

Atkins diet will help you attain good and vigorous health. The change will be felt throughout the body. Atkins nutritional approach will satisfy your nutritional requirements by allowing delicious, filling and healthy foods. It is based on the avoidance of and carb and sugars, which are usually present in junk food, which have become the life line of modern eating patterns.

Following the healthy Atkins approach you will experience more energy, lesser fatigue and higher vitality. These are all not the results of weight loss, nevertheless e the physical effects of truly dysfunctional insulin and blood sugar metabolism is strongly reversed. So during your Atkins diet, you will feel inner energy and vigorous health, even before the attainment of optimum body weight... abandoning the disastrous diet comprising of processed and refined carbohydrates, will make your body feel the real strength. Thousands of people all around the world ensure the mentioned results through their personal experience.

4. Immunity for disease resistance

This comes out to be the eventual result of vigorous body. Atkins diet plan is much like a systematic approach. It makes the body get used to low carb diet, which lead towards lower body weight. Eventually all of the issues pertaining to higher body weights are automatically eradicated. A healthy body becomes strong enough in terms of immunity to make up its own natural system of prevention against various diseases. So it is not a diet plan only, it a complete way towards healthier living.

As Atkins diet is based on least carbohydrate content in the body so insulin production is reduced to a great extent. As a result, all the related disease like diabetes, hypertension, and cardiovascular disease are largely improved.

A healthier body entails a higher quality of life. The quality of life is much more important, even more than the usual measures of beauty and attractive figure. Although weight loss is part of this diet plan, but a disease free and vigorous life will eventually make you experience the real colors of this life.

5. No reversal of result

When we talk about weight loss, one of the greatest fears people report is to regain the weight. This fear either keeps them away from putting efforts or keeps them hopeless throughout their pound-shedding venture. It is because traditional diet plans are more like an artificial medium of handling weight loss issue. It keeps the body away from energetic contents of food. The human body can sustain this condition only for a few days or maximum for few months. Just as this starvation routine is lost people start regaining. Their fear comes out to be true and this self-fulfilling prophecy never lets them attain the true weight loss condition.

In the case of Atkins diet plan, nothing is against human nature. In fact, Atkins diet isaimed at bringing back the modern human world to the natural contents present in the diet. As natural approach is followed with a steady pace so the results are permanent. These may not be sudden and spontaneous as in the case of low-fatdiets but once attained these will leave the body healthy and dynamic.

CHAPTER 3:

ATKINS DIET FAQ

Question1: Can we exclude the gram counter of fibers from the total count of carb during the Atkins diet?

Answer: Yes most experts agree to this as fiber is not involved in marinating blood sugar level it is usually not considered in weight loss counts. It does not put much impact on weight loss.

Question 2: How can we keep away from Constipation during the Atkins diet plan?

Answer: Keeping a habit of excessive water

general maintenance. If someone has an excessive problem he may need to add excessive fiber in diet including ground flaxseed, wheat bran, and psyllium husks.

Question 3: I am in the first week of Atkins plan and experiencing leg cramps, why do it is occurring? What can I do to cater this situation?

Answer: This is the phase known to be induction phase, in which there is an intense diuretic effect. Under this effect the body loses a lot of water weight, in addition to electrolytes, and minerals like calcium, magnesium, and potassium. It eventually affects the muscular breakdown and causes leg cramps. If these cramps are becoming too intense you should add salt to your salad and ask your trainer to suggest some mineral supplements.

Question 4: During Atkins diet, do I need to adjust any kind of medication?

Answer: first of all stop all the over-the-counter unnecessary medications, including cough syrup, antihistamines, antacids; diuretics sleep aids or laxatives. Other prescription medications also slow down the process of weight loss so talk to your doctor as well as Atkins guide about the situation is that both of them can decide about the best possible way. However, if you are Diabetic you need to be extra careful in taking medicine and insulin as Atkins usually lowers down the blood sugar levels. A close supervision and monitoring are needed in this case.

Question 5: do I have to cut out the consumption of vegetables during Atkins diet?

part of this myth people also consider that Atkins is all about cheese and meat consumption, which is solely a myth. Atkins poses a restriction over carbohydrates and hence starchy vegetables are inhibited which include carrots, potatoes, and beets. Based on a particular phase of Atkins diet the consumption of vegetables will vary but it is not at all absent.

Question 6: Why is Atkins diet criticized for relying too much on fat?

Answer: Actually Atkins is the only diet plan which does not restrict the intake of fats. As a result, people think that it so a kind of over-reliance on fat. But actually, Atkins involves only the intake of healthy and useful fat. Mostly monounsaturated fats present in avocado and olive oil are introduced during different phases of Atkins diet.

One of the major reasons for allowing fats is the need of fats during lowered carbohydrate intake. When the body undergoes the process of ketosis or fatburning, it makes use of fat from the food consumed as well as from the body fat.

Question 7: How much calorie count is acceptable during Atkins diet and its various phases?

Answer: The Atkins diet is based on counting the particular number of grams for carbohydrates rather than counting the calories. If you want to convert it into calories you can consider a normal range which is 1500-1800 calories, for one day, for women. In the case of men the total consumption of one day can go to 1800 - 2200 calories.

Question 8: How much carbohydrate intake is

you are, the personal carb balance is the ultimate pivotal point. You have to find out the maximum level of carbohydrate consumption which will not cause any regain your weight. But along with that, you have to consider that optimum level of carbohydrate consumption at which you feel healthy and you are able to perform daily life activities with an utmost level of vigor and energy. A little trial and error method will work out.

Question 9: Is there some Atkins diet plan to lose weight in 10 days?

Answer: Atkins diet is based upon four different phases. All of these phases are divided into various strategies and routines. It is because Atkins is believed to be the most natural approach to weight loss which makes use of the natural flexibility of human body which takes time. Once lost in a natural way, the excessive body weight never comes back. So do not try to indulge in 10 days or one week plan for weight loss.

Question 10: I have been into Atkins since last four days, and I am suffering from severe headaches. What is the reason?

Answer: The foremost reason of an excessive headache during the early days of Atkins diet is the inhibition of caffeine. Most of the people who have the habit of excessive coffee or tea drinking suffer from a headache during initial days of Atkins diet. You can go for ibuprofen to get quick relief. Some other reasons may be food sensitivities, sugar withdrawal, skipping meals, dehydration or lack of vitamins.

CHAPTER 4:

HOW TO MAXIMIZE THE CHANCES OF DIETING SUCCESS THROUGH ATKINS DIET

SUCCESS IS IN YOUR HANDS

The success of any venture is calculated through considering both the short term and long term consequences. Same is the case with the success of Atkins diet plan. Knowing about its details and consequences is no doubt a positive edge for the follower but in order to attain success, it is necessary to

Atkins diet is a fabulous diet plan but it is as good as the determination of its follower. It is nothing at its own until followed properly. Below are some points which are narrated in order to help the readers to gain the maximum benefit out of Atkins diet and enhance the chances of its success.

1. Be alert and sensitive towards food, which is at your disposal. The need for nourishment comes as the natural innate need so nature has made arrangement for the fulfillment of this need. A natural solution like seeds, meat, fowl, starch, fruits, fish and vegetables are the best solutions. Fruits and starches are the foods nature intended you to eat. On the other hand, the artificially processed and packaged Carbohydrate stuff easily available over the counters is like dead input for your body. These artificial solutions attract because of their tastes, as these are not natural and intend to seduce our taste buds.

2. Never ever ignore the presence of white flour, corn syrup and, sugar and corn starch in any of the food. No matter how less is the quantity of these ingredients, they have the capacity to ruin your efforts that you have put on Atkins diet. Always read the labels of food you consume.

During and after Atkins diet plan the healthiest solution for success is to individualize personal eating map. Try to taste new foods by increasing the assorted variety of items. The greater will be the variety of food

4. Clearly make two to three diet plans which helped you a lot in the diet session. Use them as your sacred policy of reverting back to the initial phase of success.

5. Many people achieve best results during the dieting phase but once their ideal weight is achieved they start diverting back. One way to achieve maximum benefit is to keep the consumption of alcohol and caffeine at a moderate level. Never overuse these drinks, no matter how happy are you with the immediate results of your diet plan.

6. If you have some kind of addictions, nothing can work for it, except abstinence. People only consider smoking and drugs to be part of addiction but consuming unhealthy food is itself an addiction. The temptation to get in when you pass by a fast-food restaurant can deviate you from yourdetermination. Self-denial is the only way out.

7. Exercise is not is not only related to weight loss. If you want to achieve maximum success, make exercise a routine.

8. Keep a strict check upon body composure and weight gain. Any change even the tiniest one must be handled with an utmost level of curiosity. When you keep on piling up the pounds, the reversal of result can become even more devastating.

CHAPTER 5:

THE FOUR PHASES OF ATKINS DIET

PHASE 1

(a) Induction principles for Atkins Diet

The induction phase comes out to be the most crucial of all. If this phase is not fulfilled precisely it can lead to total failure. It is therefore necessary to start with it as per the descriptions and suggestions by your Atkins diet expert.

An incorrect induction to Atkins diet will give similar result just like the ones which are achieved by any kind of traditional diet plan. All this will lead to

Here are the steps required for Phase 1 of Atkins diet plan which can also be considered as induction steps.

1. Make a routine of eating regular size meals, three times a day. Skipping meals in not recommended at all in Atkins diet. If you are awake you will not spend six hours without any intake.

2. Follow abundant consumption of protein and fat throughout the induction phase. You can go for any of the food items containing these two contents like red meat, fish, poultry, eggs and shellfish. Atkins diet also allows consumption of natural fat in the form of olive oil, mayonnaise, Butter, sunflower, vegetable oils and sunflower oil

3. Limit the consumption of carbohydrates during the first phase. In this phase make this consumption limited to just 20 grams per day you can take carbohydrates in the form of salad greens and vegetables coating higher carbohydrates. You can also consume about 3cups of salad which comes in loose packing. Or you can even change the composition even without changing the measurement of carbohydrate content. For this composition you can go for one cup of vegetables and two cups of salads.

4. Another major step to be taken in induction phase is to eradicate the consumption of bread, fruits,

cream .for the first two weeks completely eradicate the consumption of seeds and nuts. During phase 1, the diets which include the combination of carb and proteins is present, are strictly prohibited. These include legumes, kidney beans and chickpeas

5. Starvation and skipping meals is highly forbidden in Atkins diet and most importantly during the induction phase. The human body cannot resist hunger for very long and Atkins diet believes on natural processing of human body towards a healthier weight loss campaign.

6. During the induction phase start tuning up your appetite. Adjust the consumption frequency and intensity of your eating plan and frequency of meals as per the demands of your appetite. When you fell hunger signals try to consume as much as you can for satisfying your appetite. Do not indulge in ever eating. In case you do not feel any hunger signal but it has been quite some time till you have had your last meal, you can consume any snack with lowest carbohydrate content. It is because the nutritional requirement of human body cannot be ignored. Even if your body can sustain long spans without eating, it may be because of some other disorder but you have to provide the natural requirements of the body on your own.

7. While categorizing food items according to their specific composition, do not make rough or vague assumptions. If you are assuming anything to be low in

be even more precise in your measurements, which are surely a good thing, you can get access to a carb counter.

8. Do not restrict hunger in any case. Eat whenever you want to eat but by having a strict control over the particular content present in different meals. There is usually high carb content in sauces, gravies, and salad dressings. Gravy is mostly made up of cornstarch or flour or cornstarch. Salad dressings are usually composed of sugar and other high crab ingredients.

9. Always check the ingredients which are present in drink or food which you consume. Cut down the consumption of any of the product which uses aspartame as a sweetening agent. You can look up for Saccharin or Sucralose as sweetening agent. None of your consumption of these drinks should go beyond 1 gram.

10. Put a cut down at tea and coffee consumption. Any of the other drinks containing caffeine must be restricted. Higher levels of caffeine in the body lead to lower levels of sugar in the blood. As a natural inclination the body starts to carve for sugar and in that craving one forgets about any diet or determination to lose weight.

11. Enhance the water intake. In the initial phase if you are not into excessive drinking of water, make it 8 glasses of water daily. It will help you to evenly hydrate your body throughout the day and will ease you in

produced after the break down of burning fat.

12. Atkins diet also suggests ways for catering various health issues which may come in your way. Like if someone is felling constipated he can mix two tablespoons of psyllium husks in a glass of water and drink daily.

(b) Acceptable foods:

These are the food items which Atkins diet follower can eat any time and even in excessive quantity.

These include:
Fish category:
- Tuna
- Salmon
- Sole
- Trout
- Flounder
- Sardines
- Herring

Fowl category:
- Chicken
- Turkey
- Duck
- Goose
- Quail
- Pheasant

- ➢ Oysters
- ➢ Mussels
- ➢ Lobster
- ➢ Clams
- ➢ Squid
- ➢ Prawns
- ➢ Crabmeat

Meat category:
- ➢ Beef
- ➢ Lamb
- ➢ Bacon
- ➢ Veal
- ➢ Ham
- ➢ Venison

Eggs category:
- ➢ Scrambled
- ➢ Fried
- ➢ Poached
- ➢ Soft boiled
- ➢ Hard boiled
- ➢ Omelettes

Some other foods may also be considered acceptable during the first phase of Atkins diet. But you need to be careful as carbohydrate intake needs to be minimized at the best possible level. Although above categories of food are mentioned to be acceptable Atkins diet but below mentioned points are worth considering during phase 1 of Atkins diet. Processed

> Some fish items are sold in market with added sugar. These packed items will add up the carb count. Try to avoid meat and fish items which are treated with nitrates.
> Cut off from food
> Products which are not exclusively and naturally fish, meat, or fowl. These are imitations of meat food.
> Consumption of offal must not be more than 4 oz per day.

Spices

You can use all sorts of spices in Atkins diet but beware of added sugar in all sorts of spices.

Herbs

> Thyme
> Tarragon
> Sage
> Rosemary
> Pepper
> Oregano
> Ginger
> Garlic
> Dill
> Coriander
> Cayenne
> Basil

Salads

sugar content.

You can also use herbs and Lemon Juice along with spices.

You can use readymade salad Dressings only if there are without the artificial Sugar

Fats and Oils

Oils and fats are essential ingredients to be the part of our diet. Make sure to buy those with labels cold pressed.

- ➤ Olive Oil
- ➤ Canola,
- ➤ Walnut
- ➤ Soybean
- ➤ Grape seed
- ➤ Sesame
- ➤ Sunflower
- ➤ Safflower Oils
- ➤ Polyunsaturated Oils including Corn, sunflower, and Soybean Oil.

PHASE 2

ONGOING WEIGHT LOSS

With the successful induction or Phase 1, the next phase is known to be "Ongoing weight loss".

It is the phase at which one starts finding customized solutions which can fit one's special tastes. It is the best part of Atkins diet which has appeared as one of the most important reasons for its success.

- ➢ Phase 2 is considered to be a little more lenient as compared to induction, but it will surely expose the wonders by helping you in dissolving fat.
- ➢ Always show patience as the result will be gradual in their visibility and inches will drop at a slow pace. This is the ultimate beauty of Atkins diet which makes the body flexible with tiny and minute changes.
- ➢ A little intake of crabs in allowed in this phase but the quality of carbohydrates is even more important.

Principles of Ongoing weight loss phase
- ➢ Sustain fats and protein as the essential components of the nutritional plan
- ➢ Steadily enhance the daily carbohydrate intake. It should be not more than 5 grams per week
- ➢ Follow the carb ladder which is an essential part

- ➢ In the initial phase. Consume a specific food group, not more than three times in a week to start. Slowly switch it to the daily routine.
- ➢ If any of the new food items causes weight gain for you immediately stop its consumption. This phase will continue until the time you are just 5 to pounds away from your target weight.

- ➢ Carbohydrate ladder
- ➢ Excessive vegetables and salads
- ➢ Fresh cheeses
- ➢ nuts and seeds
- ➢ Berries
- ➢ Drinks low in carb
- ➢ Legumes
- ➢ Fruits except melons and berries
- ➢ Starchy veggies
- ➢ Whole grains

This ladder will be followed in the prescribed order.

PHASE 3

PRE-MAINTENANCE

This phase of Atkins diet makes you nearer to the target. You can enter this phase only after hard work, permanent determination, and healthy eating habits. These all good habits will pay you off and you will enter this phase of pre-maintenance, which is also known as the phase of permanent slimness. At Phase 3 you will only weigh 5 to 10 pounds more than your ideal weight. Entering this phase require a continuous pat on the back so that you can feel the real worth of your achievement.

> ➤ This phase is about preparing for lifetime maintenance so it needs to be carried out in a slow and start pace. Do not try to get in a hurry to achieve your goal hastily; it can destroy your entire previous struggle.
> ➤ Phase 3 is not concerned about shedding pounds; it is all about creating a program which can sustain a lifelong maintenance for the ideal weight. The weight you achieve after the whole Atkins diet will be your magic number and Phase 3 is all about keeping that magic number.

What to do?

Yin Phase 2 you had increased the carbohydrate

increase this quantity up to 10 grams a week. As you are increasing the carbohydrate intake it means that you are slowing down the pace of losing the weight.

After the initial increase at this phase, you can keep adding the carbohydrates till the point at which you feel that you are no more losing weight. If the magical number is still with you, then wait for one month or more to add more carbohydrates to the diet.

Maintain the ideal weight and monitor it closely. Accordingly add or loose carbohydrate content to diet as per your needs. It will be a point where you will reach:

Critical Carbohydrate Level for Maintenance (CCLM)

The chances of getting in trouble at this phase are higher because of these two reasons.

➤ People do not recognize that it is still about restricting and monitoring yourself. They compare it with earlier phases of Atkins, although the comparison must be with the life earlier than Atkins.

➤ People are anxious to find out that without the magnificent benefit of deep Biolysis, appetite repression has diminished.

PHASE 4

LIFETIME MAINTENANCE

This is related to the last phase and most prominent phase of Atkins. The major purposes of Phase 4 include following major intentions:

- ➤ To provide a permanent way of eating which can ensure that the follower of Atkins diet stays slim throughout the life
- ➤ To allow maximum intake of healthy carbohydrate foods, while keeping the weight within 3to 5 pounds deviation from the ideal weight.
- ➤ To prevent an addiction of foods this can be troublesome for Atkins diet by restricting the exposure to these diets.
- ➤ To teach how to revert backward to previous weight loss step ,whenever it is needed during lifetime control for weight control
- ➤ To teach about making the healthiest carbohydrate choices, this can allow a continuation to eating habits, with best levels of cholesterol and blood pressure.
- ➤ To teach about the adjustment of carbohydrate consumption during variable metabolic circumstances and changes, without allowing a weight gain
- ➤ To provide an eventual feeling of confidence and accomplishment that can spread over for

CHAPTER 6:

DRAWBACKS OF ATKINS DIET

While going on the Atkins diet you will see a number of hindrances at different point of time. It is not that simple plan, if it had been, surely everyone would have chosen it. It means it requires some extra effort, which everyone cannot put in. Rather than labeling them to be drawbacks, you can label them as challenges which one faces while following the Atkins diet. These are not out of the world challenges and one can surely treat them in one way or the other. But first

➤ **A lifelong maintenance**

If you start you inquire about the drawbacks of this diet plan from people who had been following it for many years, you will find one common answer, and i.e. lifelong maintenance is required. However, it is common for all types of weight loss diet plans. Even in the case of general wellbeing of the human body a lifelong maintenance is surely required which can make the person fed up. The best possible solution for this is to keep up the pace at a moderate level. Moreover, a continuous support and motivation system can also help you to maintain the ideal weight.

The last phase of Atkins diet is an ongoing process which will never end. It is the phase of maintenance. Many people complete first three phases with determination and motivation but in the case of the last phase, they feel that they cannot continue anymore. This has been reported as the biggest drawback of Atkins diet.

➤ **Hunger signals are reduced**

In the case of Atkins diet, the reduction in carbohydrate intake and a steady pace of weight loss eventually make you accustomed to it. Most of the people report that they encounter reduced hunger pangs in the case of Atkins diet. They think that they will lose the overall energy. But if you will follow the Atkins diet in real terms your body will never feel devoid of energy and overall wellbeing. Keeping a

signals your body will not feel lethargic or out of energy.

> ### ➤ A close observation on diet is required

As Atkins diet is a low carbohydrate diet, it means that one needs to be alert about the intake of his or her food. You cannot eat straightaway; you need a closer observation on each and every label of food packaging. Even in some cases you will need a carb counter. It is a little bit demanding, especially in the case of hectic work routines or if you are having kids. But this drawback can be surely covered. The initial few days of carb count and detailed observation make you well aware about the quantity of a particular diet and its related carb counter. The initial few days spent well enough, pay you back and you start feeling aware about your day to day meal.

CHAPTER 7:

COMMON MISTAKES MADE IN ATKINS DIET AND HOW TO AVOID THEM

Atkins diet is a long way to go so people sometimes indulge in some deviating behaviors as they lose focus throughout this long span. It is, therefore, necessary to mention some of the mistakes which are most commonly pursued during various phases of

your energies in a completely opposite and negative direction. Some of the biggest ones are mentioned here:

Being scared of Fat

The human body requires dietary fat in order to stimulate the proper burning of body fat. Natural fats are not any hazard for the body when a controlled amount of carb is taken in. whenever you take a snack made of carb; try to add some protein or fat with it. One simple example is to consume cheese accompanied with cucumber slices.

Consuming Hidden Carbs

One the first day of your Atkins diet make a promise with yourself not to consume anything without reading the package labels over any of the food item you consume. It will help you a great way for avoiding sneaky Carbs and other added sugar. If a packet of food item claims to be low in calorie count, it doesn't entail lower carbohydrate content. Do not get a victim of hidden carb by eating low-calorie diet. Low calorie does not always entail low carbohydrates so you can get a victim of fallacy. Moreover consume full fat packaging for salad dressings, mayonnaise, salad dressing and the like. Low-fat packaged foods always contain added sugar in order to replace the extra flavor of the excessive oil. In case some label is not readable, you can go for Carb Counter so there is no need for taking a risk for any count.

Choosing the incorrect Products

inconvenience is to use low-carb products which are labeled with Atkins title. These labeled diets have been researched extensively in order to make sure that the effect on the blood sugar level is minimal. You can also get special diets for every phase of Atkins.

Counting continuously for Total Carbs and ignoring the Net Carbs

As going through this book you have become well aware of the fact that carbohydrate and its correct count are most critical to the success of this plan. Now the major mistake usually done is considering the incorrect way of counting. There are two measures, one is total carb count which denotes the whole number of carbohydrates in grams taken in. the other is net carb count which excludes the grams of fibers from the total carb. It is because fiber is not related to any of the impactson your blood sugar. All other sugar substitutes need to be counted in this count. If you have a carb allowance for a day or a week, do not substitute it with low fiber diet, starches or sugar. On the other hand, do not try to shun away carbohydrates all at once. Depending upon the phase you have to consume the right number of carbohydrates.

Eating all salt-free:

Although a lot of salts will be surely devastating for you but in the case of normal blood circulation and other chemical activities taking place in the human body, one surely needs to get a proper amount of salt. It will also keep you away from headaches leg cramps

CHAPTER8:

RECIPES

PHASE 1 RECIPES

Breakfast Recipes

1. BASQUE EGGS WITH TOMATOES AND HAM

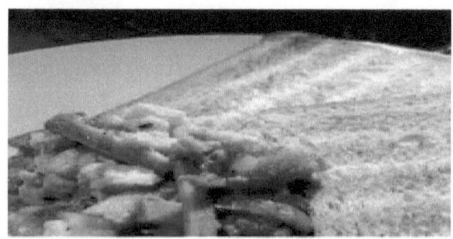

Ingredients:

- ➢ Olive Oil (Extra Virgin)- 3 tbsp

- ➢ Onions- 1 medium

- ➢ Bell Peppers (Roasted)- 8 oz

- ➢ Red Tomatoes -2 plums

- ➢ Basil- 5 1/2 tbsp

- ➢ Cayenne Pepper- 1/4 tsp

- ➢ Eggs (Whole)- 12 large

- ➢ Butter Stick (Unsalted)- 6 tbsp

- ➢ Fresh Ham- 6 oz

- ➢ Garlic- 3 tbsp

Directions:

Use medium heat to boilingoil. Use a large skillet. Now in this oil add onions along with garlic and cook for five to six minutes. Now mix tomatoes, peppers, and cayenne. Place the lid over the pan and cook for 10 minutes. When you will uncover the pan you will see a thick sauce, let it simmer. Add pepper and salt. Whisk eggs in another pan. Use melted butter to cook eggs. Mix with simmering sauce and eat while medium hot.

2. Cinnamon waffles in buttermilk

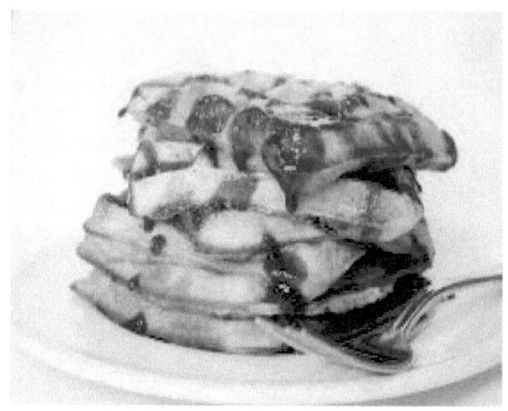

Ingredients:

➢ Soy Flour (Whole Grain)- 1 cup

➢ Sucralose Based Sweetener - 2 tbsp

➢ Cinnamon- 2 tbsp

➢ Baking Powder - 3 tbsp

➢ Baking Soda- 1/2 tsp

➢ Buttermilk - 3/4 cup

➢ Butter Stick (Unsalted)- 6 tbsp

➢ Whole Eggs - 3 large

➢ Vanilla Syrup (Sugar-Free)- 1 1/2 oz

➢ Tap Water- 1/2 cup

➢ Cooking Spray (Original Canola)

given over the packet. Mix together, sugar substitute, soy flour, cinnamon, baking soda and baking powder. Now mix buttermilk, eggs, butter, and syrup. Continue stirring until you see a well-blended batter. Mix cold water to make the batter easily spreadable and spoonable. Use oil Spray for a waffle iron. Fill waffle with already prepared batter. Cook as per instructions are given on packet.

3. Hazelnut chocolate smoothie

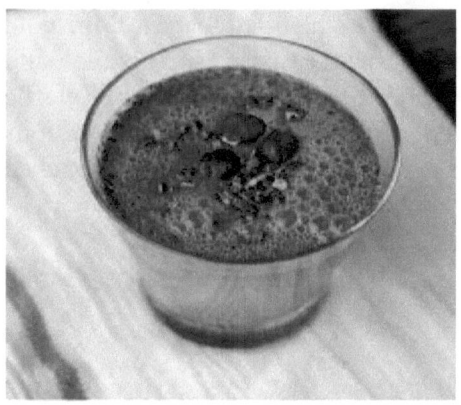

Ingredients:
- Chocolate Whey Protein- 2 scoops

- Heavy Cream- 1 tbsp

- Hazelnut Syrup (Sugar-Free)- 12 tbsp

Directions:
Put cream, protein mix and syrup in your electric blender. Add ice as per your preference of chilliness. Blend well until smooth. Sprinkle with finely ground cinnamon.

4. Portobello broilers in Chicken

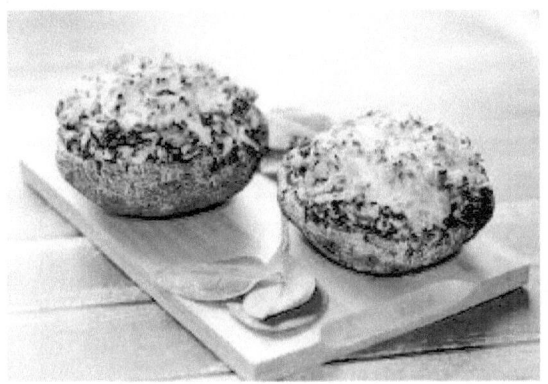

Ingredients:

- ➤ Eggs (Whole)- 4 large

- ➤ Chicken Breast- 8 oz

- ➤ Spring Onions (chopped)- 3 tbsp

- ➤ Olive Oil (Extra Virgin)- 2 tbsp

- ➤ Mushroom Caps (Portobello)- 6 caps

- ➤ Salt- 1/4 tsp

- ➤ Black Pepper- 1/4 tsp

- ➤ Italian Seasoning- 1/4 tsp

- ➤ Mozzarella Cheese - 1/4 cup

Directions:

Prepare the broiler by preheating for ten minutes. Make vertical thin slices of chicken breast. Use medium flame for heating oil and cooking breast pieces with mushrooms by placing on a baking sheet and sprinkling pepper, salt and herbs. Put in oven for ten minutes. Now place chicken egg mixture over mushrooms. Add melted cheese over top.

5. Salsa eggs

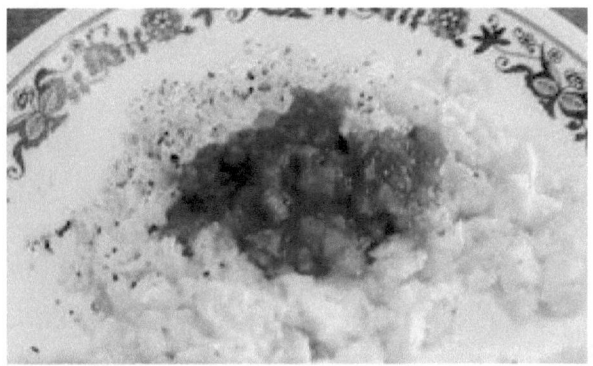

Ingredients:
- California Avocados (skinless)- 1/2 fruit

- Salsa- 1 oz

- Eggs (Whole)- 2 large

Directions:
Cook eggs by suing a few drops of virgin olive oil. Use a small skillet and a medium flame. Flip each side of the egg, one after the other. Sprinkle pepper and salt. Now transfer in serving the dish and place a layer of salsa followed with avocado slices.

Lunch Recipes

6. BagnaCauda

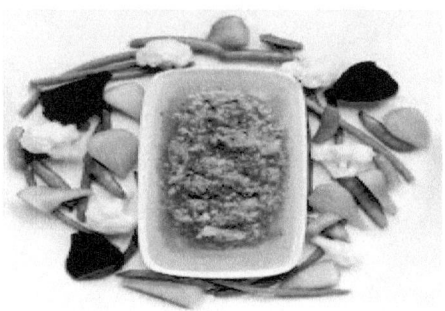

Ingredients:
- ➢ Olive Oil(Virgin)- 1/2 cup

- ➢ Butter Stick (Unsalted)- 1/4 cup

- ➢ Garlic- 3 tbsp

- ➢ Anchovy - 8 anchovies

Directions:
Take up a small saucepan to heat the olive oil along with butter. Make sure that the heat is not too high. In that mixture put anchovies and garlic. Cook them all, quite gently for 10 minutes. Cool till you smell garlic fragrance. Now add pepper and serve hot with vegetables.

7. Eggplant puree

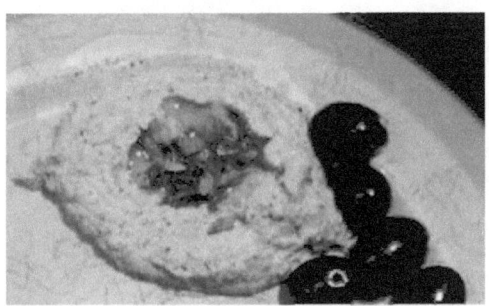

Ingredients:

- Eggplant- 1 lb

- Olive Oil (Virgin)- 3/4 cup

- Garlic- 2 tbsp

- Parsley- 1 tbsp

- Salt- 1/8 tsp

- Black Pepper- 1/8 tsp

Directions:

You will need a preheated microwave oven at around 425°F. Prepare the eggplant by cutting through all of the sides with profound slashes. Now put the pieces over the baking pan. Bake until eggplant turns soft. It will need around 30 minutes. Keep the baked eggplant aside and wait till it becomes cool. Now Peel off the skin and put in an electric processor. Add oil parsley and garlic in a blender and cheap. Add pepper to taste.

8. Goat cheese and tomato dip

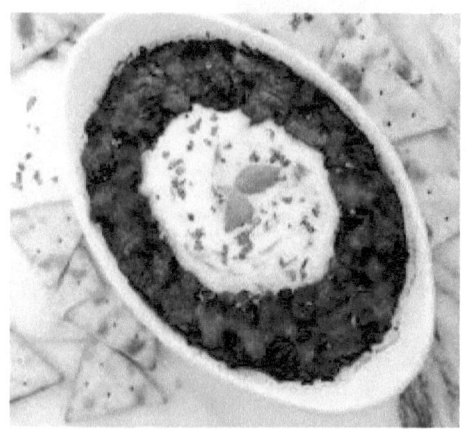

Ingredients:
- Cream Cheese- 4 oz
- Goat Cheese - 4 oz
- Sour Cream - 1/3 cup
- Sun-Dried Tomatoes- 3/4 cup
- Bell Peppers (Roasted)-3 oz
- chopped Onions- 1/4 cup
- Jalapeno Peppers- 2
- Garlic- 1/2 tsp
- Cilantro (Coriander)- 1/8 cup

Directions:
Mix the goat cheese, softened cream cheese, and

yellow onion and garlic. Mix well to join. Add up salt and fresh black pepper. Keep this mixture for 8 hours in the refrigerator. Serve fresh vegetables with this mixture. You can use this mixture for around two weeks if refrigerated.

9. Coconut bread in low Carbs

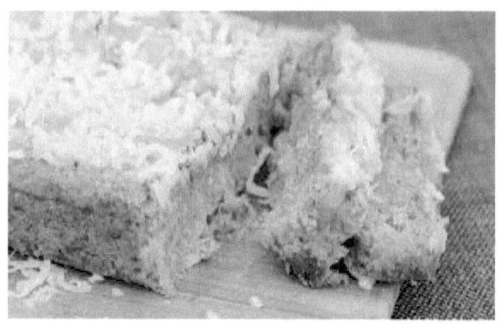

Ingredients:

➢ Eggs (Whole)- 6 large

➢ Butter Stick (Unsalted)- 1/2 cup

➢ Xylitol- 1 tsp

➢ Coconut Flour- 3/4 cup

➢ Baking Powder (Double Acting, Straight Phosphate)- 1 tsp

➢ Salt- 1/2 tsp

Directions:

Prepare your oven at 350°F. Take a bread pan and grease with oil. Mix eggs melted butter and xylitol. Gently whisk for two minutes. Mix together baking powder, coconut flour, and salt. Now add eggs to the flour mixture and merge until thickened. Cook for 35 to 40 minutes. Upon proper cooking, the sides will pull away along the pan. The color will turn to golden brown.

Let the mixture cool down for 10 minutes then

10. Peppermint chocolate truffle

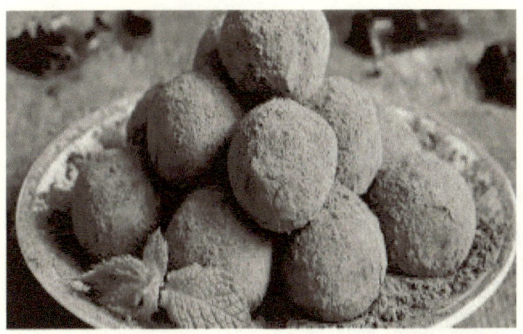

Ingredients:
- Chocolate Chips (Sugar-Free)- 4 oz

- Heavy Cream- 2 tbsp

- Butter Stick (Unsalted)- 1 tbsp

- Peppermint Candy (Sugar-Free)- 10

- Vanilla Extract- 1 tbsp

Directions:
Put chocolate in a microwavable bowl and leave it aside. Take another microwavable bowl to mix butter and cream. Keep it aside too. Now put the chocolate bowl in oven firstly for 30 seconds on medium heat and then for 20 seconds on high heat.

Dinner Recipes

11. Roasted beef and lettuce wrap

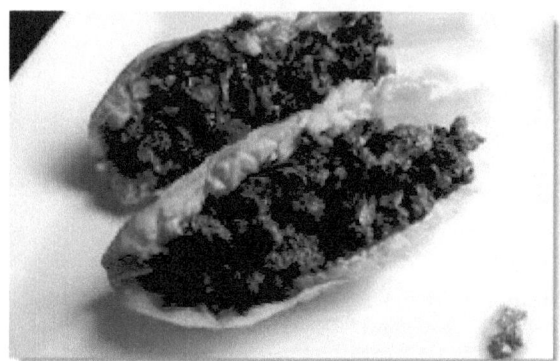

Ingredients:

➢ Roast Beef- 4 oz boneless

➢ Provolone Cheese - 2 oz

➢ Red Sweet Pepper- 1/4 medium

➢ Romaine Lettuce - 2 leaf

➢ Real Mayonnaise - 1 tbsp

➢ Horseradish Sauce- 1/8 tbsp

Directions:

Cut out the bottom part of lettuce leaves. Place them flat on a washed surface. Now place a cheese slice over each. Mix garlic powder and mayonnaise. Add garlic up to taste. Add pepper and salt. Now spread this mixture over cheese slices. Over this cheese layer place roasted beef. Make a thin strip of bell pepper and keep toothpick to firmly tighten up the role.

12. Baked Tofu

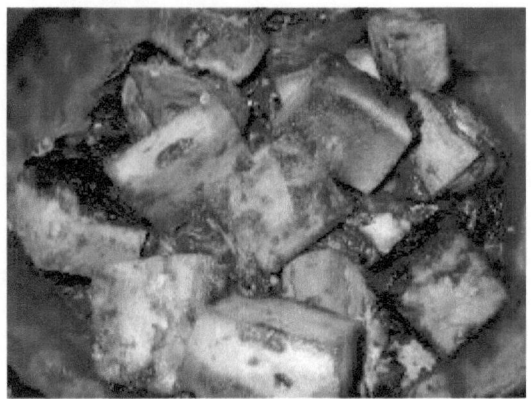

Ingredients:
- Silken Tofu - 6 oz
- Chipotle Marinade - 1 serving

Directions:
Drain out tofu and use a paper towel with a paper towel. Make equal sized strips. Use Chipotle Marinade to marinate this mixture for 45 minutes. Separate from the marinade and prepare oven at 375°F. Take a flat pan and use a brush for greasing it evenly. Put tofu over the pan and bake for 10 minutes. Turn the sides till bath sides become crispy.

13. Tuna Salad

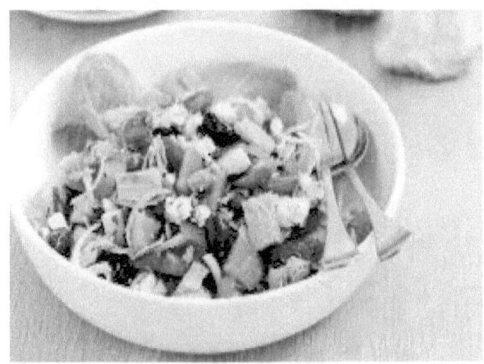

Ingredients:
- Tuna (Canned)- 6 oz

- Lemon Juice - 1 oz

- Real Mayonnaise- 3 tbsp

- Arugula (Rocket)- 2 cups

- Slice Cucumber (with Peel)- 1/2 cup

- Olive Oil- 1 tbsp

Directions:
Take a small bowl and mix together tuna, zest, lemon juice and mayonnaise. Evenly sprinkle black pepper and salt through the mixture. Now Serve it with cucumber and arugula and pour olive oil.

Snacks Recipes

14. Kale chips

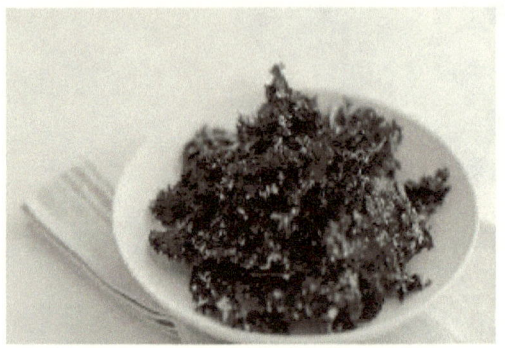

Ingredients:

➢ Kale- 7 oz

➢ Olive oil- 1 tbsp

➢ Dash salt- 1/8

Directions:

Prepare your oven at 250°F. Make two separate baking sheets using parchment paper. Drain out Kale stalks and separate the leaves. Evenly place the stalks over kitchen boards. Use a kitchen scissor to make bite-sized pieces of kale leaves. Evenly toss the kale leaves with olive oil. It is better to toss by hand. Sprinkle sea salt as per taste. Now place these leaves over baking dish and bake for thirty minutes. Bake till the leaves turn crispy. Save in air tight container.

15. Grilled cheese Bread

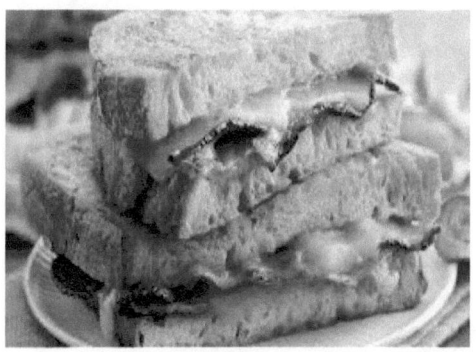

Ingredients:
- Cheddar Cheese- 1/4 cup
- Tomatoes- 2 slices
- Butter Stick - 1 tsp
- Atkins Cloud Bread - 1 serving

Directions:
Use medium heat to boilingoil. Use a large skillet. Now in this oil add onions along with garlic and cook for five to six minutes. Now mix tomatoes, peppers, and cayenne. Place the lid over the pan and cook for 10 minutes. When you will uncover the pan you will see a thick sauce, let it simmer. Add pepper and salt. Whisk eggs in another pan. Use melted butter to cook eggs. Mix with simmering sauce and eat while medium hot.

PHASE 2

Breakfast

16. Cinnamon Pie Crust

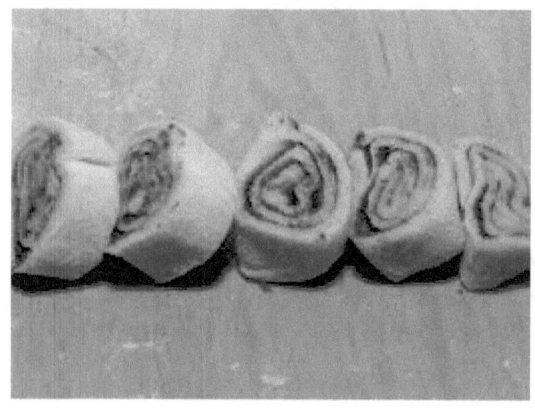

Ingredients:
- Salt- 1/4 tsp

- Sweetener (Sucralose Based)- 1 tsp

- Cinnamon- 1 tsp

- Butter Stick- 1/2 cup

- Baking Mix (Low-Carb)- 3 3/4 servings

- Tap Water- 2 tbsp

Directions:
Mix together, sugar substitute, soy flour, cinnamon, baking soda and baking powder. Now mix buttermilk, eggs, butter, and syrup. Continue stirring until you see a

waffle iron. Fill waffle with already prepared batter. Cook as per instructions are given on packet.

17. Almond Pancakes

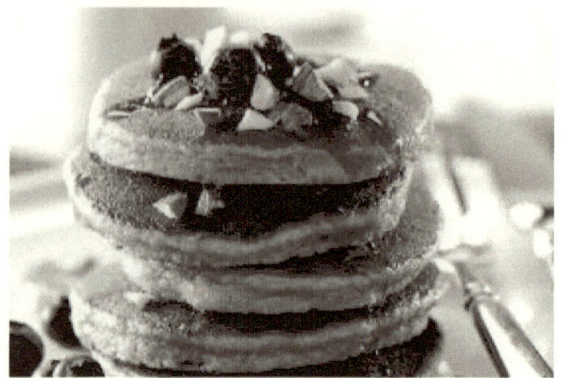

Ingredients:

➤ Whey Protein- 2 oz

➤ Almond Flour- 1/4 cup

➤ Soy Flour- 3 tbsp

➤ Baking Powder (Double Acting)- 1 tbsp

➤ Cottage Cheese- 1/3 cup

➤ Eggs (Whole)- 3 large

Directions:

Cook eggs by suing a few drops of virgin olive oil. Use a small skillet and a medium flame. Flip each side of the egg, one after the other. Sprinkle pepper and salt. Now transfer in serving the dish and place a layer of salsa followed with cottage slices.

18. Atkins Waffles

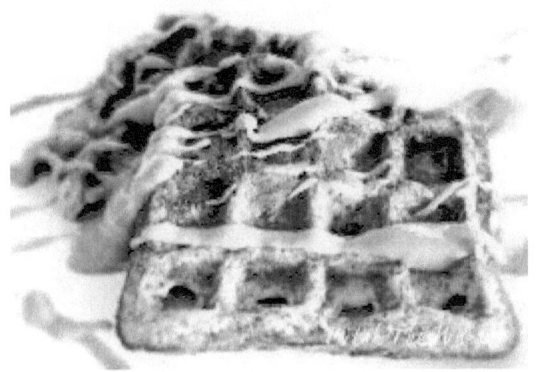

Ingredients:

➤ Sugar Substitute (Sucralose Based)- 1 packet

➤ Egg (Whole)- 1 large

➤ Baking Powder -2 tbsp

➤ Salt- 1/4 tsp

➤ Cream -1 cup

➤ Baking Mix (Low-Carb)- 3 servings

Directions:

Prepare the broiler by preheating for ten minutes. Make vertical thin slices of chicken breast. Use medium flame for heating oil and cooking breast pieces with onion. Continue cooking for five minutes. Now add whisked eggs and keep stirring. Side by side prepare mushrooms by placing on a baking sheet and sprinkling pepper, salt and herbs. Put in oven for ten minutes. Now place chicken egg mixture over mushrooms. Add

19. Basque eggs

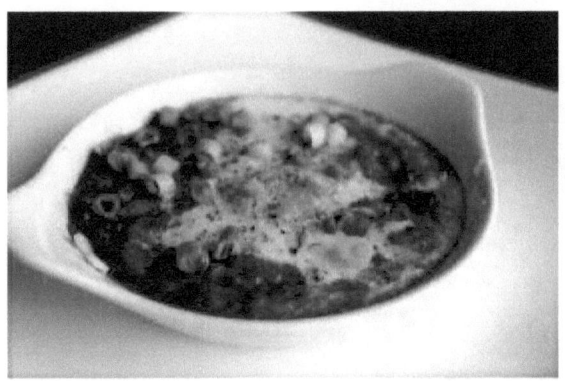

Ingredients:

➢ Olive Oil-3 tbsp

➢ Onions- 1 medium

➢ Bell Peppers- 8 oz

➢ Red Tomatoes- 2

➢ Basil- 5 1/2 tbsp

➢ Cayenne Pepper- 1/4 tsp

➢ Eggs (Whole)- 12 large

➢ Butter Stick- 6 tbsp

➢ Fresh Ham- 6 oz

➢ Garlic- 3 tbsp

Directions:

Cook eggs by suing a few drops of virgin olive oil

Now transfer in serving the dish and place a layer of salsa followed with cottage slices.

20. Beef with green pepper

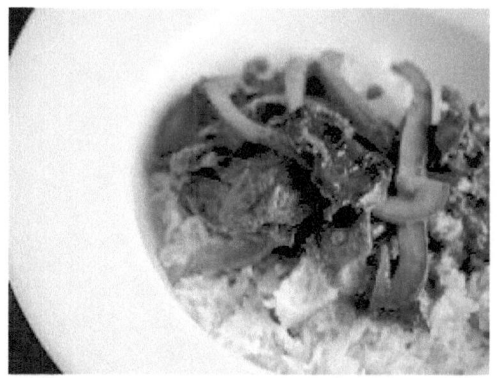

Ingredients:
- chopped Onions- 1/4 cup

- Olive Oil- 1 tbsp

- Sweet Pepper- 1/2 cup

- Cheddar Cheese- 1/2 cup

- Ground Beef - 5 oz

Directions:
Prepare the broiler by preheating for ten minutes. Make vertical thin slices of chicken breast. Use medium flame for heating oil and cooking breast pieces with onion. Continue cooking for five minutes. Now add whisked eggs and keep stirring. Side by side prepare mushrooms by placing on a baking sheet and sprinkling pepper, salt and herbs. Put in oven for ten minutes. Now place chicken egg mixture over mushrooms. Add melted cheese over top.

Lunch

21. Coconut muffin

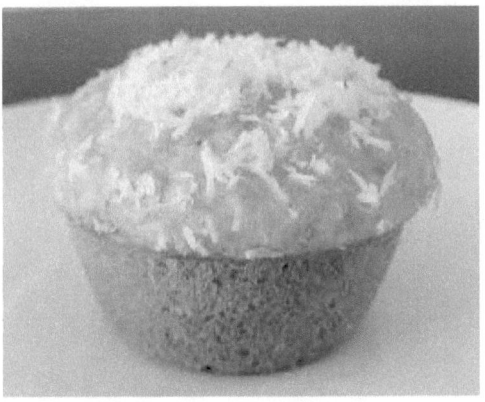

Ingredients:

➤ Meal Flour- 1/8 cup

➤ Coconut Flour- 1/3 tbsp

➤ Cinnamon- 1/2 tsp

➤ Baking Powder (Double Acting, Straight Phosphate)- 1/4 tbsp

➤ Salt- 1/8 tsp

➤ Egg (Whole)- 1 large

➤ Olive Oil- 1/3 tbsp

Directions:

First of all make waffle iron with the instructions given over the packet. Mix together, sugar substitute, soy flour, cinnamon, baking soda and baking powder. Now mix buttermilk, eggs, butter, and syrup. Continue

spoonable. Use oil Spray for a waffle iron. Fill waffle with already prepared batter. Cook as per instructions are given on packet.

22. Tuna kebabs

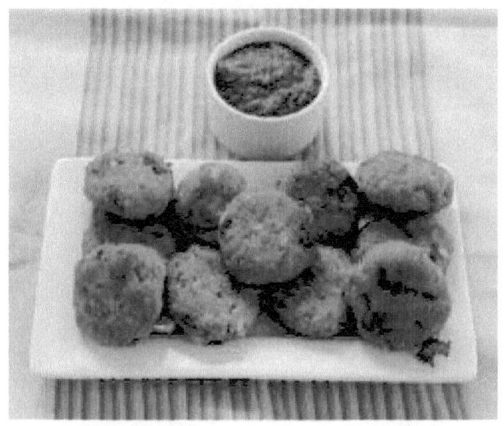

Ingredients:
- Soy Sauce (Gluten Free)- 5 1/3 tbsp
- Rice Wine- 2 2/3 floz
- Sesame Oil- 1 tbsp
- Ginger- 1 tbsp
- Garlic- 3 tbsp
- Sugar Substitute- 2 tbsp
- boneless Tuna- 3 large
- Spring Onions- 3 large
- Red Sweet Pepper- 1 large
- Eggplant- 3/4 lb

and grease with oil. Gently whisk for two minutes. Mix together baking powder, coconut flour, and salt. Now add eggs to the flour mixture and merge until thickened. Cook for 35 to 40 minutes. Upon proper cooking, the sides will pull away along the pan. The color will turn to golden brown.

Let the mixture cool down for 10 minutes then shift to a wire rack to finish cooling for 30 minutes. Now put in an air-tight container.

23. Leek and asparagus soup

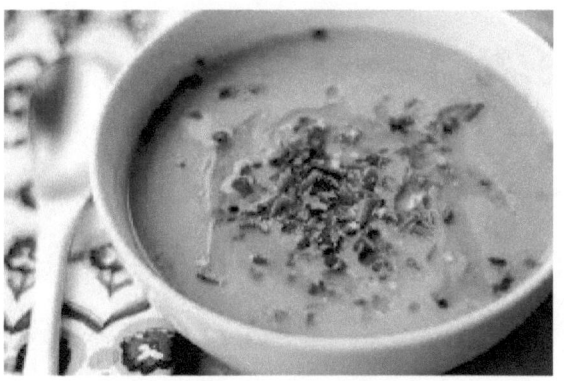

Ingredients:
- ➢ Butter Stick- 2 tbsp

- ➢ Leeks- 1 leek

- ➢ Asparagus- 3/4 lb

- ➢ Garlic- 1 tsp

- ➢ Chicken Broth - 14.5oz

- ➢ Heavy Cream- 1/3 cup

Directions:
Prepare the broiler by preheating for ten minutes. Make vertical thin slices of chicken breast. Use medium flame for heating oil and cooking breast pieces with onion. Continue cooking for five minutes. Now add whisked eggs and keep stirring. Side by side prepare mushrooms by placing on a baking sheet and sprinkling pepper, salt and herbs. Put in oven for ten minutes. Now place chicken egg mixture over mushrooms. Add melted cheese over top.

24. Atkins brownies

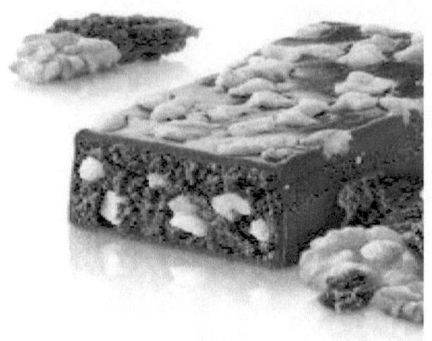

Ingredients:

- ➢ Chocolate Squares (Unsweetened)- 4 oz

- ➢ Heavy Cream- 1/2 cup

- ➢ Eggs- 5 large

- ➢ Sugar Substitute- 1 cup

- ➢ Butter Stick- 1/2 cup

- ➢ Baking Powder (Double Acting, Straight Phosphate)- 2 tbsp

- ➢ Baking Mix- 4 1/2 serving

Directions:

Prepare your oven at 350°F. Take a bread pan and grease with oil. Mix eggs and melted butter. Gently whisk for two minutes. Mix together baking powder, coconut flour, and salt. Now add eggs to the flour mixture and merge until thickened. Cook for 35 to 40 minutes. Upon proper cooking, the sides will pull away

shift to a wire rack to finish cooling for 30 minutes. Now put in an air-tight container.

25. Zucchini soup

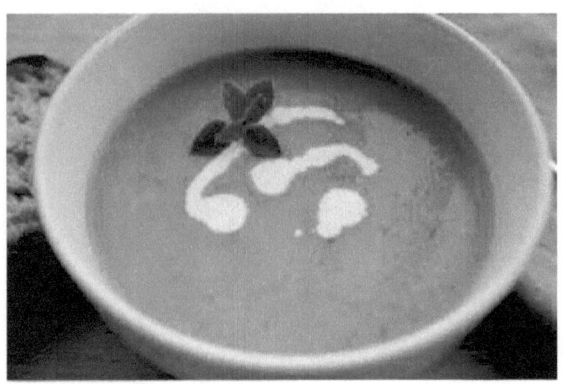

Ingredients:

- California Avocado- 1

- Olive Oil-2 tbsp

- (Spring Onions- 4 medium

- Ginger- 1 tsp

- Garlic- 1 clove

- Zucchinis- 2 medium

- Vegetable Broth- 29 oz

- Tap Water- 1 cup

- Salt- 1/2 tsp

Directions:

Prepare the broiler by preheating for ten minutes. Make vertical thin slices of chicken breast. Use medium

whisked eggs and keep stirring. Side by side prepare mushrooms by placing on a baking sheet and sprinkling pepper, salt and herbs. Put in oven for ten minutes. Now place chicken egg mixture over mushrooms. Add melted cheese over top.

Dinner

26. Garlic toast

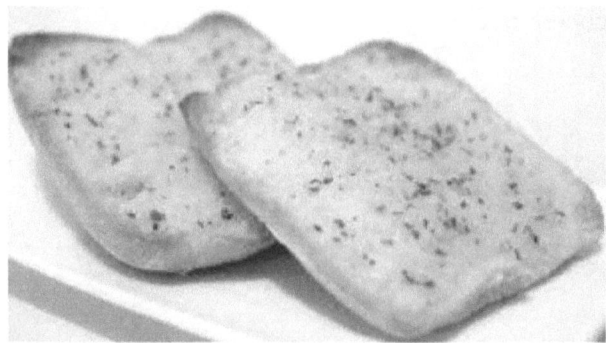

Ingredients:

➢ Olive Oil- 1/4 cup

➢ Garlic- 1 oz

➢ Soy Flour (Whole Grain)- 2 cups

➢ Baking Powder -3 tbsp

➢ Eggs -2 large

➢ Salt- 1/2 tsp

➢ Club Soda- 1/2 can

Directions:

Mix together eggs, soy flour, cinnamon, baking soda and baking powder. Now mix buttermilk, eggs, butter, and syrup. Continue stirring until you see a well-blended batter. Mix cold water to make the batter easily spreadable and spoonable. Use oil Spray for a waffle

27. Chicken puffs

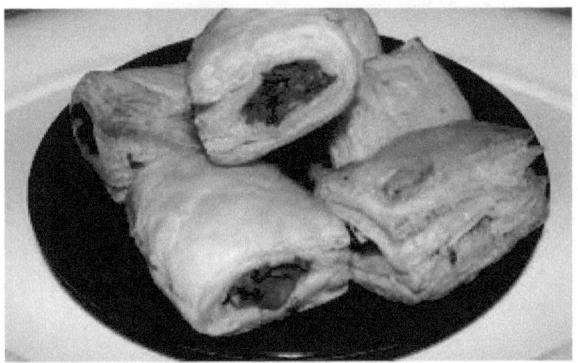

Ingredients:
- Chili Powder- 2 tbsp

- Cayenne Pepper- 1 tsp

- Yellow Mustard Seed- 2 tbsp

- Salt- 2 tbsp

- Baking Mix (Low-Carb)-1/2 serving

- Chicken Wing- 32 oz

Directions:
Prepare the broiler by preheating for ten minutes. Make vertical thin slices of chicken breast. Use medium flame for heating oil and cooking breast pieces with onion. Continue cooking for five minutes. Now add whisked eggs and keep stirring. Side by side prepares mushrooms by placing on a baking sheet and sprinkling pepper, salt and herbs. Put in oven for ten minutes. Now place chicken egg mixture over mushrooms. Add melted cheese over top

28. Coconut macaroons

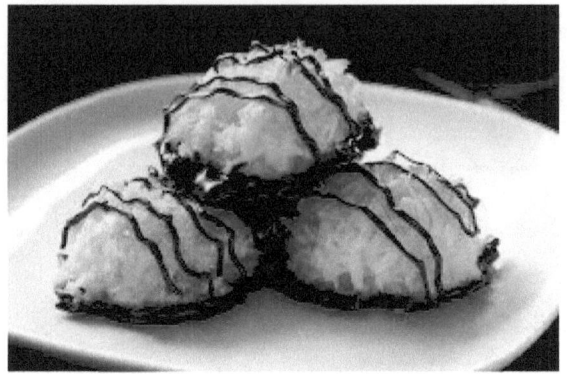

Ingredients:
- ➢ Cooking Spray- 1/3 second
- ➢ Egg Whites- 4 large
- ➢ Sweetener (Sucralose Based)- 2/3 cup
- ➢ Vanilla Extract- 1/2 tsp
- ➢ Salt- 1/4 tsp
- ➢ Dried Coconut- 2 cups

Directions:
Use medium heat to boilingoil. Use a large skillet. Now in this oil add onions along with garlic and cook for five to six minutes. Now mix tomatoes, peppers, and cayenne. Place the lid over the pan and cook for 10 minutes. When you will uncover the pan you will see a thick sauce, let it simmer. Add pepper and salt. Whisk eggs in another pan. Use melted butter to cook eggs. Mix with simmering sauce and eat while medium hot.

Snacks

29. Almond pretzels

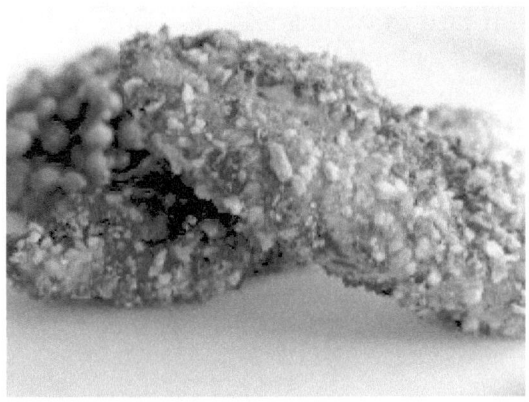

Ingredients:
- ➢ Baker's Yeast -1 1/2 tbsp

- ➢ Tap Water- 2 tbsp

- ➢ Almond Flour- 1 1/2 cups

- ➢ Salt- 1/8 tsp

- ➢ Baking Powder (Straight Phosphate)- 3/4 tsp

- ➢ Guar Gum- 1/4 tsp

- ➢ Red Pepper (Flakes)- 1/4 tsp

- ➢ Black Pepper- 1/4 tsp

- ➢ White Pepper- 1/4 tsp

- ➢ Egg (Whole)- 1 large

- ➤ Egg White- 1 large

- ➤ Kosher Salt- 1 tsp

Directions:

Use medium heat to boilingoil. Use a large skillet. Now in this oil add onions along with garlic and cook for five to six minutes. Now mix tomatoes, peppers, and cayenne. Place the lid over the pan and cook for 10 minutes. When you will uncover the pan you will see a thick sauce, let it simmer. Add pepper and salt. Whisk eggs in another pan. Use melted butter to cook eggs. Mix with simmering sauce and eat while medium hot.

30. White bean puree

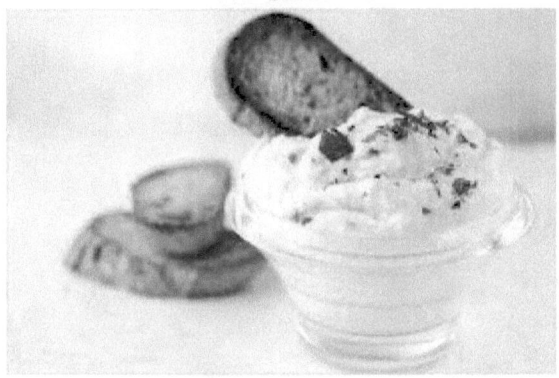

Ingredients:
- Olive Oil- 1 tbsp

- Garlic- 2 cloves

- Rosemary - 1 tsp

- Cannellini Beans- 2 cups

- Salt- 1/2 tsp

- 1/8 tsp Black Pepper

Directions:
Take up a small saucepan to heat the olive oil along with butter. Make sure that the heat is not too high. In that mixture put anchovies and garlic. Cook them all, quite gently for 10 minutes. Cool till you smell garlic fragrance. Now add pepper and serve hot with white beans.

PHASE 3

Breakfast

31. Protein pancakes

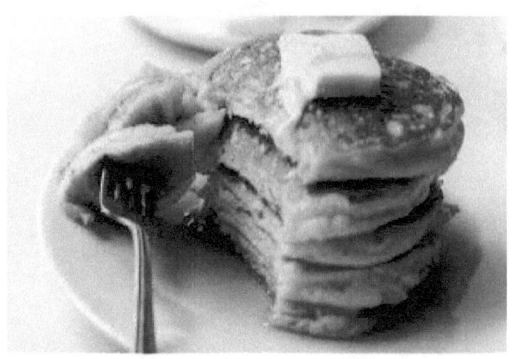

Ingredients:
- Whey Protein- 2 oz
- Meal Flour- 1/4 cup
- Soy Flour- 3 tbsp
- Baking Powder - 1 tbsp
- Cottage Cheese- 1/3 cup
- Eggs (Whole)- 3 large

Directions:
Cook eggs by suing a few drops of virgin olive oil. Use a small skillet and a medium flame. Flip each side of the egg, one after the other. Sprinkle pepper and salt. Now transfer in serving the dish and place a layer of

32. Breakfast Peppers

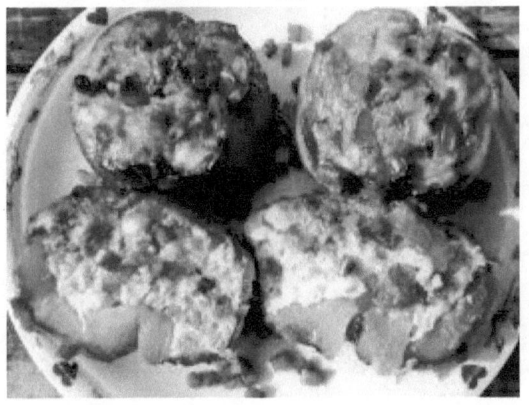

Ingredients:
- Beef Chorizo- 4 oz
- Ground Beef - 4 oz
- chopped Onions- 1/2 cup
- Cheddar Cheese- 1/4 cup
- Eggs (Whole)- 3 large
- Red Peppers- 2 medium

Directions:
Take out and use butter and cream mixture as a pouring over the moderately melted chocolate. Let it simmer for sit 5 minutes. Blend well to make a smooth mixture. If you feel that chocolate is forming lumps heat it for another 2 seconds. When the mixture gets moderately low to temperature, place the bowl in the fridge. Form balls of small size and roll in cocoa powder and peppermint candies. Place over a serving dish.

33. Cheddar Omelette

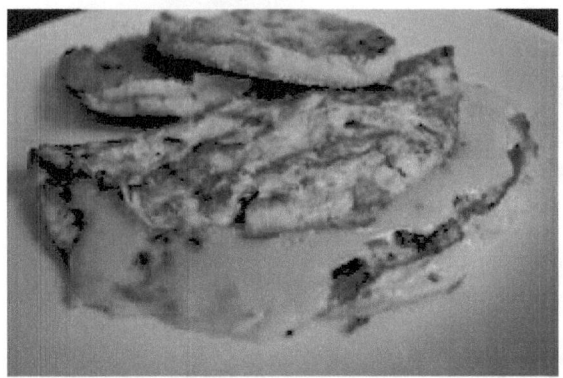

Ingredients:
- Beef Chorizo- 4 oz

- Ground Beef - 4 oz

- Onions- 1/2 cup

- Cheddar Cheese- 1/4 cup shredded

- Eggs - 3 large

- Red Peppers- 2 medium

Directions:
Cook eggs by suing a few drops of virgin olive oil. Use a small skillet and a medium flame. Flip each side of the egg, one after the other. Sprinkle pepper and salt. Now transfer in serving the dish and place a layer of salsa followed with cheese slices.

34. Chicken Portobello

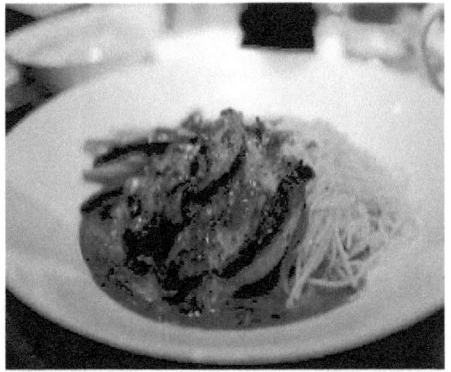

Ingredients:

- Eggs - 4 large

- Chicken Breast- 8 oz

- Spring Onions- 3 tbsp

- Olive Oil- 2 tbsp

- Mushroom Caps- 6 caps

- Salt- 1/4 tsp

- Black Pepper- 1/4 tsp

- Italian Seasoning- 1/4 tsp

- Mozzarella Cheese -1/4 cup

Directions:

Cook mushroom caps by suing a few drops of virgin olive oil. Use a small skillet and a medium flame. Flip each side of the egg, one after the other. Sprinkle

35. French casseroles

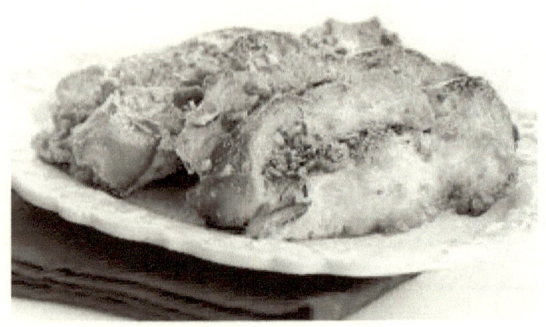

Ingredients:
- Eggs - 14 large
- Butter Stick (Unsalted)- 10 tbsp
- Coconut Flour- 1 cup
- Baking Powder -1 1/2 tbsp
- Salt- 3/4 tsp
- Heavy Cream- 1 cup
- Coconut Milk (sugar-free)- 1 cup
- Cinnamon- 1 tsp
- Nutmeg -1/4 tsp
- Flavoured Syrup- 1/2 cup

Directions:
Mix together, sugar substitute, soy flour, cinnamon, baking soda and baking powder. Now mix buttermilk, eggs, butter, and syrup. Continue stirring until you see a well-blended batter. Mix cold water to make the batter easily spreadable and spoonable. Fill roles with already prepared batter. Cook as per instructions are given on packet.

Lunch

36. Sesame Seed Beef

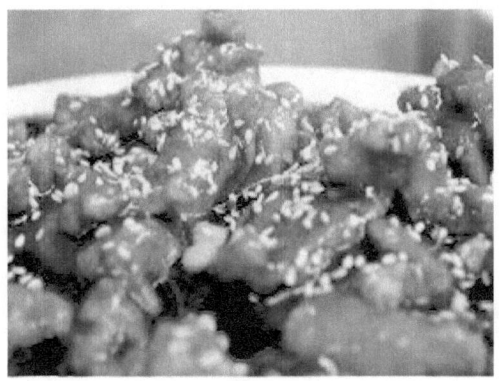

Ingredients:
- Garlic- 1/4 tsp

- Soybean Sauce- 1/2 tbsp

- Rice Vinegar (sugar and sodium free- 1/8 tbsp

- Sesame Oil- 1/4 tsp

- Curry Powder- 1/8 tsp

- Ginger (Ground)- 1/16 tsp

- Mix Salad- 1 cup

- Vegetable Oil- 1/2 tbsp

- Red Peppers- 1/4 large

Make vertical thin slices of beef. Use medium flame for heating oil and cooking breast pieces with onion. Continue cooking for five minutes. Now add whisked eggs and keep stirring. Side by side add mushrooms by placing on a baking sheet and sprinkling pepper, salt and herbs. Put in oven for ten minutes.

37. Lobster salad

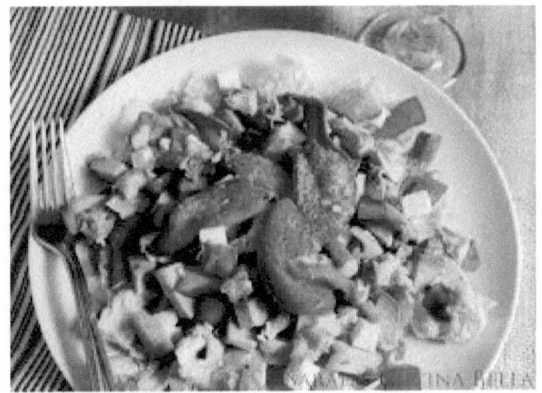

Ingredients:

- Northern Lobster- 3/4 lb

- Chinese Cabbage - 2 cups

- Red Pepper- 1/2 small

- Spring Onions- 4 medium

- Sesame Seeds- 1 tbsp

- Rice Vinegar- 2 tbspSodium

- Soybean Sauce- 2 tbsp

- Vegetable Oil- 1 tbsp

- Sesame Oil- 1 tbsp

- Ginger- 1 tbsp

Directions:

Take a small bowl and mix together Spring Onions,
Sesame Seeds, Ginger and red pepper. Evenly sprinkle

38. Atkins Meatballs

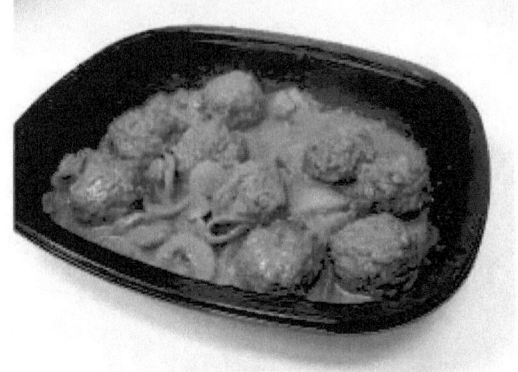

Ingredients:
- ➤ Olive Oil- 1 tbsp

- ➤ Spring Onion- 1/2 large

- ➤ Garlic- 1 1/2 tbsp

- ➤ Ground Veal- 1/2 lb

- ➤ Ground Beef -1/2 lb

- ➤ Parmesan Cheese - 1/2 cup

- ➤ Eggs -2 large

- ➤ Salt- 1/2 tsp

- ➤ Black Pepper- 1/4 tsp

Directions:
Prepare the broiler by preheating for ten minutes. Make vertical thin slices of beef. Use medium flame for heating oil and cook with onion. Continue cooking for five minutes. Now add whisked eggs and keep stirring.

39. AtkinsPizza

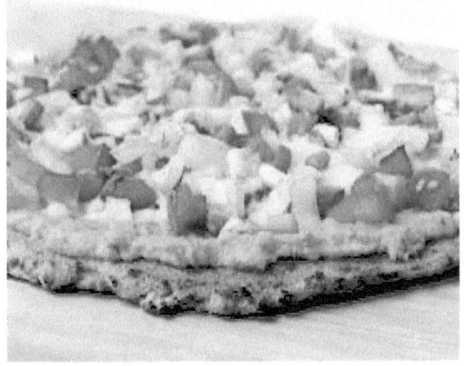

Ingredients:

➢ Baking Powder - 1 1/2 tbsp

➢ Salt- 1/2 tsp

➢ Tap Water- 1 1/8 cups

➢ Olive Oil- 3 tbsp

➢ Mozzarella Cheese - 1 cup

➢ Chicken Breast- 8 oz

➢ Sweet Pepper- 1/2 medium

➢ Red Onion- 1 small

➢ Barbecue Sauce- 4 servings

Directions:

Take out and use butter and cream mixture as a pouring over the moderately melted chocolate. Let it simmer for sit 5 minutes. Blend well to make a smooth mixture. If you feel that chocolate is forming lumps

40. Mustard-basil sauce

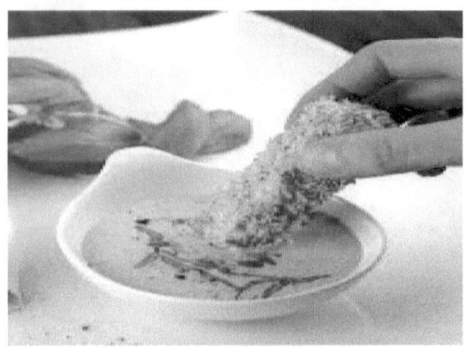

Ingredients:

- Atlantic Cod- 2 lbs

- Basil- 16 tbsp

- Garlic- 3 tbsp

- Oregano- 1 tbsp

- Olive Oil- 7 tbsp

- Lemon Juice- 1/4 cup

- Atkins Bread- 4 servings

- Dijon Mustard- 2 tbsp

Directions:

Mix together Dijon Mustard, eggs, oregano and lemon juice. Continue stirring until you see a well blended batter. Mix cold water to make the batter easily spreadable and spoonable. Fill waffle with already prepared batter. Cook as per instructions given on packet.

Dinner

41. Atkins Muffin

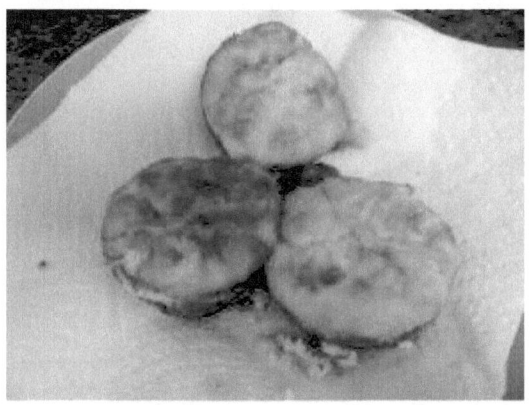

Ingredients:

- ➤ Meal Flour- 1/4 cup

- ➤ Baking Powder - 1/4 tsp

- ➤ Salt- 1/8 tsp

- ➤ Cinnamon- 1/2 tsp

- ➤ Egg (Whole)- 1 large

- ➤ Vegetable Oil- 1 tbsp

Directions:

Mix buttermilk, eggs, butter and syrup. Continue stirring until you see a well-blended batter. Mix cold water to make the batter easily spreadable and spoonable. Use oil Spray for meal flour. Fill waffle with

42. Cauliflower fritters

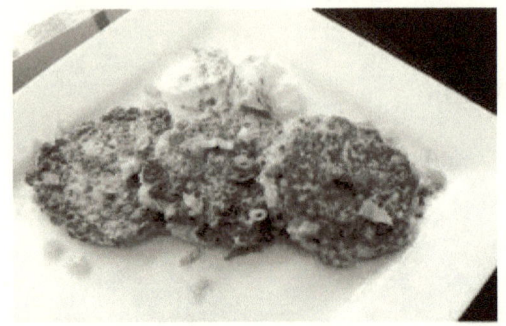

Ingredients:

➤ Cauliflower- 1/2 head

➤ Greek Yogurt- 1/3 cup

➤ Baking Powder -

➤ Salt- 1/4 tsp

➤ White Pepper- 1/4 tsp

➤ Cumin- 1/4 tsp

➤ Coriander Seed- 1/4 tsp

➤ Nutmeg (Ground)- 1/8 tsp

➤ Egg Whites- 3 large

➤ Olive Oil- 1 tbsp

➤ Coconut Flour (High Fiber)- 2 tbsp

Directions:

Cook eggs by suing a few drops of virgin olive oil. Use a small skillet and a medium flame. Flip each side of coconut flour one after the other. Sprinkle pepper

43. Pistachio cookies

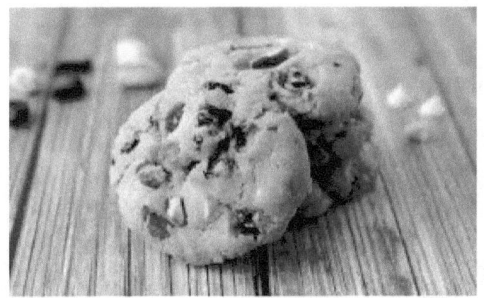

Ingredients:
- Pistachio Nuts - 1/2 cup
- Oatmeal- 1/4 cup
- Wheat Flour- 1/3 cup
- Soy Flour- 1/3 cup
- Salt- 1/8 tsp
- Baking Powder -1/4 tsp
- Butter Stick- 1/2 cup

Directions:
Put butter sticks in a microwavable bowl and leave it aside. Take another microwavable bowl to mix baking powder and pistachio nuts. Keep it aside too. Now put butter bowl in oven firstly for 30 seconds on medium heat. Sprinkle additional pistachio nuts.

Snacks

44. Lime-coconut mousse

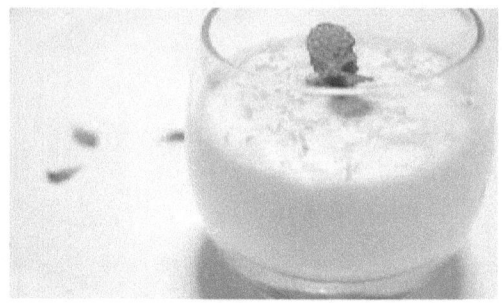

Ingredients:

- ➤ Cream Cheese- 1/4 cup

- ➤ Fresh Lime Juice- 1/4 cup

- ➤ Vanilla Extract- 1 tsp

- ➤ Heavy Cream- 1 cup

- ➤ Coconut powder- 1 tbsp

Directions:

Gently mix cream and cheese in a bowl to make a frothy liquid. Now mix coconut powder. Mix this froth in fresh lime. Enjoy chilled.

45. Creamy Feta Salad

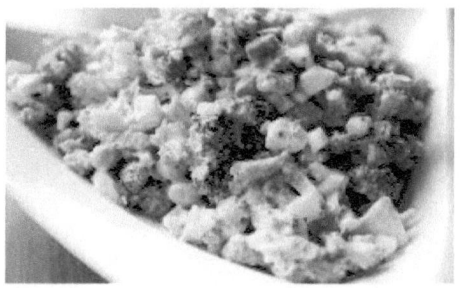

Ingredients:
- Cucumber – 2 large
- Red Onion- 1/4 medium
- Red Tomatoes- 1 large
- Kalamata Olives- 2 oz
- Feta Cheese- 1/4 cup
- Peppermint - 4 tbsp
- Olive Oil- 6 tbsp
- Wine Vinegar- 2 tbsp

Directions:

Mix all the ingredients well and pour vinegar to form a perfect salad. You can also add any vegetable depending upon the calorie and carb content.

PHASE 4

Breakfast

46. Breakfast Burrito

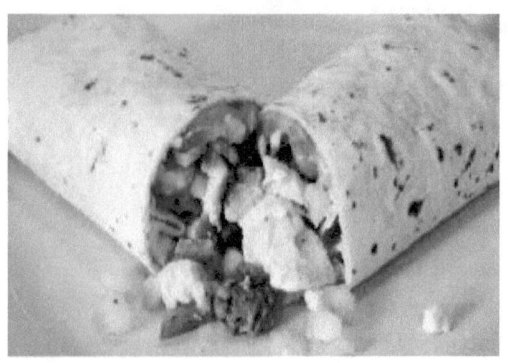

Ingredients:

- Salt- 1/2 tsp

- Cayenne Pepper- 1/4 tsp

- Vegetable Oil- 1 tbsp

- Eggs (Whole)- 4 large

- Red Peppers- 3 tbsp

- Spring Onions- 2 tbsp

- Pepper- 1

- Tortillas (Low Carb)- 2

- Tabasco Sauce- 1/8 tsp

- Salsa- 2 oz

Directions:

Cook eggs by suing a few drops of virgin olive oil. Use a small skillet and a medium flame. Flip each side of the egg, one after the other. Sprinkle pepper and salt. Now transfer in serving the dish and place a layer of salsa followed with Tobacco sauce.

47. Carrot Latkes

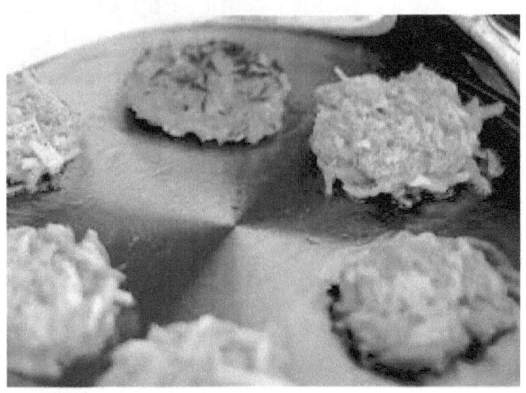

Ingredients:

- Zucchini- 12 oz

- Salt- 3/4 tsp

- Carrots- 5 medium

- Onion- 1 small

- Eggs (Whole)- 4 large

- Black Pepper- 1/2 tbsp

- Vegetable Oil- 1/2 cup

- Cuisine Bread- 1 1/2 servings

Directions:

Prepare the broiler by preheating for ten minutes. Make vertical thin slices of chicken breast. Use medium flame for heating oil and cooking breast pieces with onion. Continue cooking for five minutes. Now add pepper, salt and herbs. Put in oven for ten minutes. Now place chicken egg mixture over mushrooms. Add melted cheese over top

48. Cloud bread

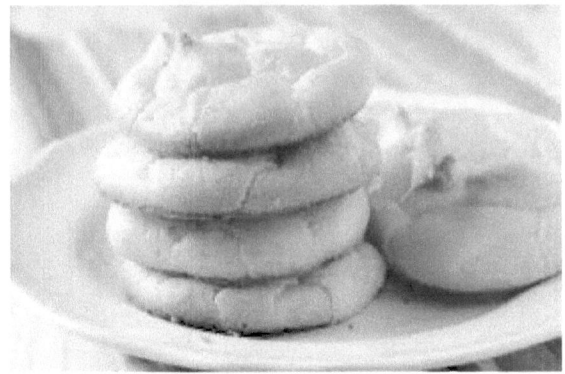

Ingredients:
- Eggs- 2 large
- Heavy Cream- 2 tbsp
- Cinnamon- 1/4 tsp
- Nutmeg (Ground)- 1/8 tsp
- Cloud Bread- 3 servings

Directions:
Put cream, protein mix and syrup in your electric blender. Add nutmeg and ice as per your preference. Blend well until smooth. Sprinkle with finely ground cinnamon.

49. Crust-lessQuiché

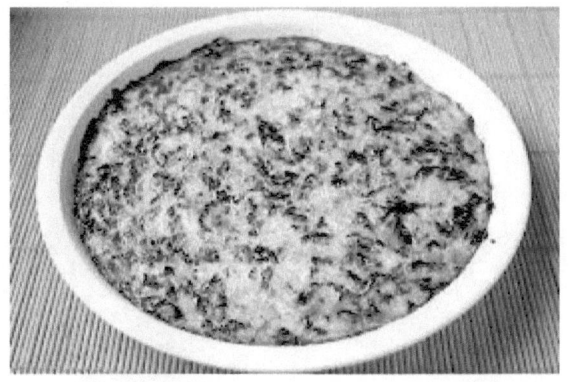

Ingredients:
- Olive Oil- 1 tbsp
- Cheddar Cheese- 1 cup
- Tap Water- 1/2 cup
- Thyme- 1/4 tsp
- Leaf Oregano- 1/4 tsp
- Salt- 1/2 tsp
- Eggs - 4 large
- Black Pepper- 1/4 tsp
- Rosemary - 1/4 tsp
- Flower Clusters- 1 lb
- Onion- 1/2 small

Directions:

mixture put clusters and rosemary. Cook them all, quite gently for 10 minutes. Cool till you smell garlic fragrance. Now add pepper and serve hot with vegetables.

50. Spinach egg

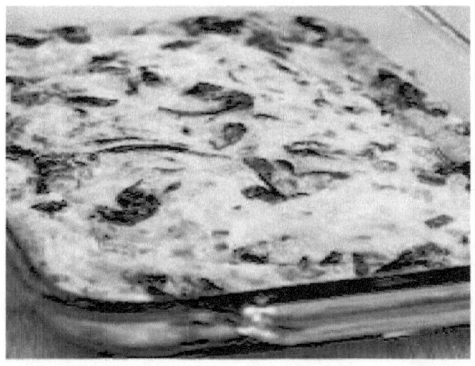

Ingredients:

➢ Vegetable Oil- 1 tbsp

➢ Baby Spinach- 2 1/16 cups

➢ Eggs - 2 large

➢ Feta Cheese- 1/2 oz

Directions:

Cook eggs by suing a few drops of virgin olive oil. Use a small skillet and a medium flame. Flip each side of the egg, one after the other. Sprinkle pepper and salt. Now transfer in serving dish and place a layer of salsa followed with avocado slices.

Lunch

51. Apricot Brisket

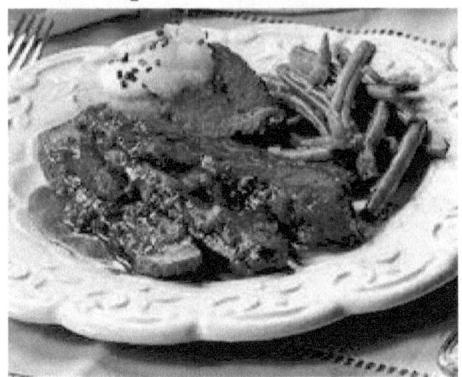

Ingredients:
➤ Beef Brisket -4 lbs

➤ Salt- 2 tbsp

➤ Paprika- 2 tbsp

➤ Black Pepper- 1 tbsp

➤ Apricot Preserves- 3 tbsp

Directions:
Take up a small saucepan to heat the olive oil along with butter. Make sure that the heat is not too high. In that mixture put beef and garlic. Cook them all, quite gently for 10 minutes. Cool till you smell garlic fragrance. Now add pepper and serve hot with apricot preserves.

52. Peas and Mushrooms

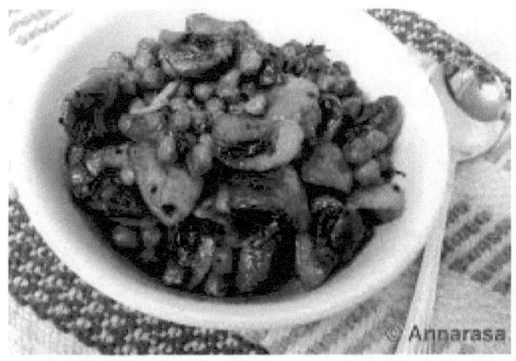

Ingredients:

- ➤ Butter Stick- 3 tbsp

- ➤ Spring Onions- 3 medium

- ➤ Garlic- 1 tbsp

- ➤ Mushroom Cap- 3oz

- ➤ Vinegar - 1/4 cup

- ➤ Tap Water- 1 cup

- ➤ Asparagus- 1 lb

- ➤ Green Peas- 1/2 cup

Directions:

Mix tomatoes, peppers, and cayenne. Place the lid over the pan and cook for 10 minutes. When you will uncover the pan you will see a thick sauce, let it simmer. Add pepper and salt. Whisk eggs in another pan. Use melted butter to cook eggs. Mix with simmering sauce

53. Bacon wrap

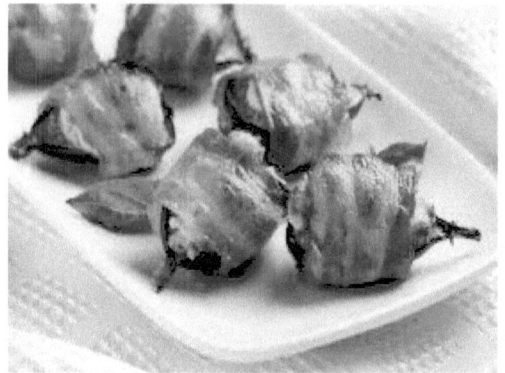

Ingredients:

➤ Eggs- 2

➤ Real Mayonnaise- 1 tbsp

➤ Yellow Mustard- 1 packet

➤ Original Flatbread- 1

➤ Turkey Bacon- 1 1/2 oz

Directions:
Prepare the broiler by preheating for ten minutes. Make vertical thin slices of chicken breast. Use medium flame for heating oil and cooking breast pieces with onion. Continue cooking for five minutes. Now add whisked eggs and keep stirring. Side by side add mushrooms by placing on a baking sheet and sprinkling pepper, salt and herbs. Put in oven for ten minutes. Now place chicken egg mixture over mushrooms. Add melted cheese over top

54. Cauliflower Risotto

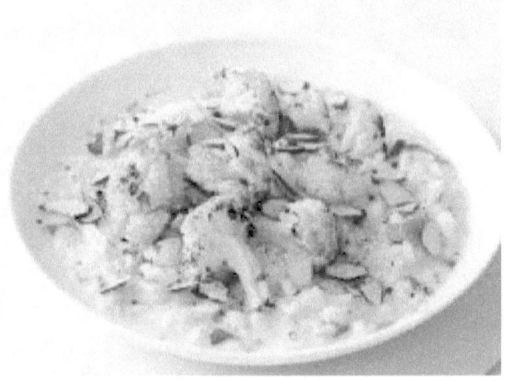

Ingredients:

➤ Butter Stick- 3 tbsp

➤ Spring Onions- 3 medium

➤ Garlic- 1 tbsp

➤ Mushroom Cap- 3oz

➤ Vinegar - 1/4 cup

➤ Tap Water- 1 cup

➤ Cauliflower- 1flower

Directions:

Mix garlic powder and mayonnaise. Add garlic up to taste. Add pepper and salt. Now spread this mixture over cheese slices. Over this cheese layer place roasted beef. Make a thin strip of bell pepper and keep adding layers over beef. Now roll it in such a way that you start at the end of pepper. Roll firmly and use a toothpick to firmly tighten up the role.

55. Cheese Soufflé

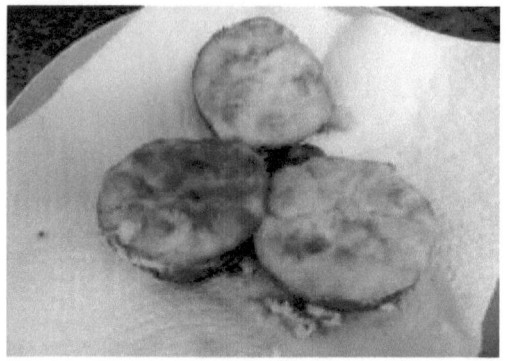

Ingredients:

- ➢ Eggs - 6 large

- ➢ Butter Stick- 1/4 cup

- ➢ Soy Flour- 2 tbsp

- ➢ Pastry Flour- 1/8 cup

- ➢ Heavy Cream- 3/4 cup

- ➢ Tap Water- 3/4 cup

- ➢ Cheddar Cheese- 2 cups

- ➢ Salt- 1/4 tsp

- ➢ Cayenne Pepper- 1/8 tsp Red

Directions:

Mix heavy cream and pastry flour. Add cheese up to taste. Add pepper and salt. Now spread this mixture over cheese slices. Over this cheese layer place roasted

Dinner

56. Tortilla wraps

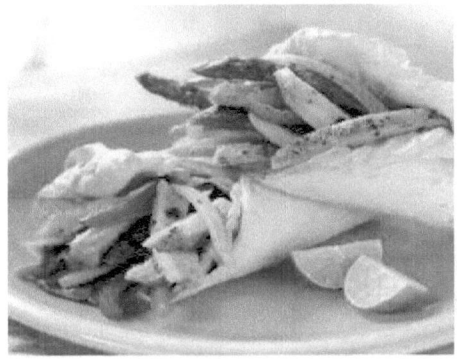

Ingredients:
- Coconut Flour- 3 tbsp

- Chili Powder- 3/4 tsp

- Salt- 1/8 tsp

- Egg - 3 large

- Coconut Milk (Unsweetened)- 1/2 cup

- Olive Oil- 1 1/3 tbsp

Directions:
Prepare the broiler by preheating for ten minutes. Make vertical thin slices of chicken breast. Continue cooking for five minutes. Now add whisked eggs and keep stirring. Add mushrooms by placing on a baking sheet and sprinkling pepper, salt and herbs. Put in oven for ten minutes. Now place chicken egg mixture over

57. Atkins Fish fillets

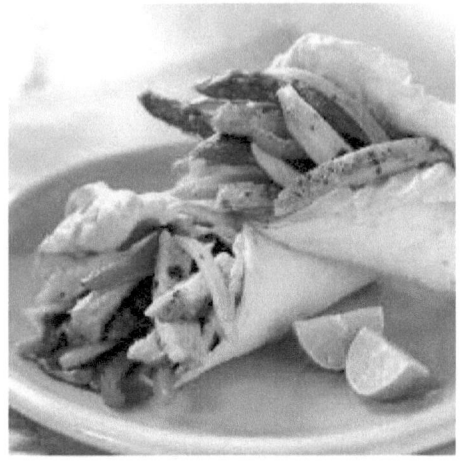

Ingredients:

➢ Sesame Oil- 4 tbsp

➢ Garlic- 1 1/2 tbsp

➢ Chicken Broth -1 1/2 cups

➢ Ginger- 4 tbsp

➢ Rice Vinegar (sodium free) -2 tbsp

➢ Soybean Sauce- 2 tbsp

➢ Channel Catfish - 2 lbs

Directions:

Cook eggs by suing a few drops of virgin olive oil. Use a small skillet and a medium flame. Flip each side of the egg, one after the other. Sprinkle pepper and salt. Now transfer in serving the dish and place a layer of cooked fish followed with avocado slices.

58. Chocolate butter Haystacks

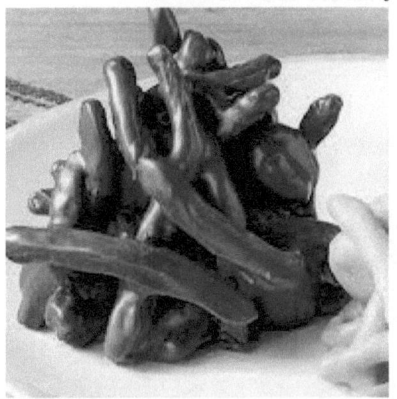

Ingredients:
➢ Butter Stick- 2 tbsp

➢ Cocoa Powder - 3 tbsp

➢ Stevia- 1 pinch

➢ Salt- 1/16 tsp

➢ Peanut Butter - 1/4 cup

➢ Flaked Coconut (Unsweetened)- 2 cups

Directions:
Take up a small saucepan to heat the butter sticks. Make sure that the heat is not too high. In that mixture put anchovies and garlic. Cook them all, quite gently for 10 minutes. Cool till you smell garlic fragrance. Now add pepper and serve hot with peanut butter.

Snacks

59. Ham Rollups

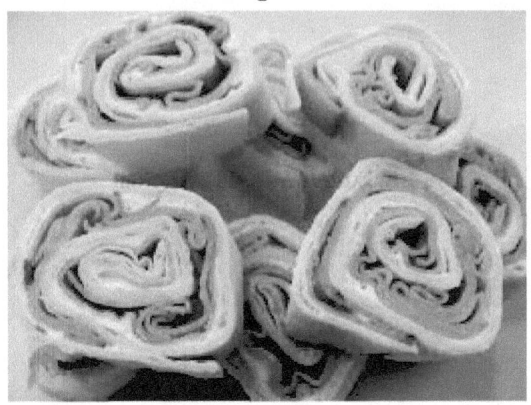

Ingredients:
- ➢ Yam bean- 2 oz

- ➢ Ham (cooked)- 2 oz

- ➢ Jack Cheese – 1 oz

- ➢ Aioli- 1 serving

Directions:
Cook eggs by suing a few drops of virgin olive oil. Use a small skillet and a medium flame. Flip each side of the egg, one after the other. Sprinkle pepper and salt. Now transfer in serving the dish and place a layer of salsa followed with avocado slices.

60. Cheddar black olives

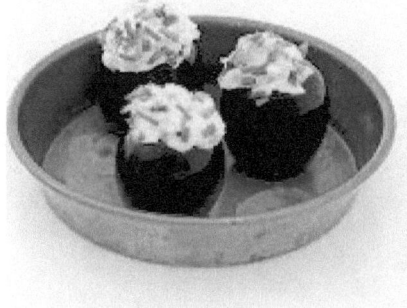

Ingredients:
- ➢ Black Olives (Greek)- 7

- ➢ Cheddar Cheese - 1 oz

Directions:
This is the simplest recipe. All you have to do put the need of a spoon inside the hole of olive to make it bigger. Fill with cheddar cheese and enjoy.

CHAPTER 9:

SAMPLE MEAL PLAN FOR INDUCTION PHASE

Apart from the recipes here is a sample plan for your fits week of Atkins diet. Based on this sample you can make meal plans for rest of the week. Even changes and alterations in this plan are possible based on your individual needs. Consult with your Atkins trainer before following any plan, especially for the first week.

SHOPPING LIST FOR WEEK 1:

Before you proceed to the meal plan for the first week, it is essential to get hold of all the necessary items which are required for this meal plan. All these items need to be readily available so that you can carry along according to the nutrients necessary for human body so that you can maintain a good balance of all the related nutrients.

Fats:
➢ Olive oil

Vegetables:
➢ Basil
➢ Broccoli
➢ Cauliflower
➢ Celery
➢ Snap Peas
➢ Onions
➢ Mixed Greens
➢ Hass Avocados
➢ Green or Red Bell Peppers
➢ Cucumbers
➢ Spinach
➢ Tomatoes
➢ Vegetables:
➢ Zucchini

Atkins Products:
➢ Atkins Bars
➢ Atkins Frozen Meals
➢ Atkins Shakes
➢ Atkins Treats

Proteins:
➢ Bacon
➢ Bone-in Pork Chop
➢ Chicken Breasts
➢ Eggs
➢ Ground Beef

MEAL PLAN FOR WEEK 1

Meal plan for the first week comprises of variable carbohydrate count so you need to follow it in the mentioned way. Each day comprises of a different setup and categorization of food items so that you may not get bored out of it.

Day 1: Monday

Zucchini- 1 small

Cheddar- 1½ oz

3.2g Net Carbs

2.6g FV

Frozen Crust-less

Chicken Pot-Pie

mixed greens - 1 cup

Italian dressing (creamy)- 1 cup

1g Net Carbs

0g FV

Strawberry Shake (Atkins)

1g Net Carbs

0g FV

Broccoli florets- 1 cup

Hollandaise Sauce- 2 Tbsp

mixed greens- 2 cups

Italian dressing (creamy)- 1 cup

4.7g Net Carbs

4.3g FV

Delight Shake in Milk Chocolate (Atkins style)

3.2g Net Carbs

2.6g FV

Chocolate Chip Granola Bar (Atkins Meal)

3g Net Carbs

0g FV

Bell pepper (green, sliced)- 1 cup

Ranch Dressing- 2 Tbsp

3.6g Net Carbs

2.7g FV

Atkins frozen chicken

Broccoli Alfredo

Mixed greens- 1½_cups

Italian dressing (creamy)- 2 tbsp

7.4g Net Carbs

4g FV

DAY 3 WEDNESDAY:

Vanilla shake (Atkins style)

1g Net Carbs

0g FV

Swedish Meatballs (Atkins Frozen)

2g Net Carbs

0g FV

Coconut Almond Delight (Atkins Delight)

2.0g Net Carbs

0g FV

Whitefish (fillet)- 6 oz

Broccoli florets- 2 cups

Herb-butter blend- 1 tbsp

Hass avocado- ½

Italian dressing- 2 tbsp

7.9g Net Carbs

7.1g FV

DAY 4 THURSDAY:

½cup chopped

red bell pepper

3.8 g Net Carbs

3g FV

Bacon- 1 slice

Blue cheese dressing- 2 tbsp

Chicken breast- 6 oz

Diced Monterey- ¼_ cup

Hass avocado- ½_

Jack cheese

Medium tomato- ½_

Mixed greens- 1 cup

5.7g Net Carbs

4.6g FV

Coconut Almond Delight (Atkins Delight)

2.0g Net Carbs

0g FV

Broccoli florets- 2 cups

Herb-butter blend- 1 tbsp

Hass avocado- ½

Italian dressing- 2 tbsp

7.9g Net Carbs

7.1g FV

Day 5 FRIDAY:

Caramel shakes (Atkins cafe)

3g Net Carbs

0g FV

Chocolate Peanut Butter Bar (Atkins Meal)

2g Net Carbs

0g FV

Sliced cucumber- ¾cup

Greek Vinaigrette- 2 Tbsp

3.3g Net Carbs

3g FV

Crustless Chicken Pot Pie (Atkins Frozen)

broccoli florets- 1 cup

olive oil- 1 Tbsp

6.6g Net Carbs

3.9g FV

DAY 6 SUNDAY:

Cranberry Almond Bar(Atkins Daybreak)

2g Net Carbs

0g FV

Canned tuna- 4 oz

Mayonnaise- 2 tbsp

Snap peas(chopped)- ½ cup

Bell pepper (red)- ¼_ cup

Tomato- 1 medium

7.2g Net Carbs

7.2g   FV

Atkins Vanilla shake

1g Net Carbs

0g FV

Ground beef- 6 oz

Crumbled- 1 tbsp

Blue cheese

Zucchini- 1 medium

Olive oil- 1 tbsp

Hass avocado- ½

Slice tomato- ½_ inch

6.6g Net Carbs

3.9g FV

DAY 7 SATURDAY:

Cherry tomatoes- 5

Mozzarella cheese (fresh)- 2 oz

Olive oil- 1 tbsp

Fresh basil - 1 tbsp

2.3g Net Carbs

2.3g FV

Sesame Chicken Stir-Fry (Atkins Frozen)

7g Net Carbs

2.2g FV

Chocolate Peanut Nougat Bar (Atkins Snack)

2.0g Net Carbs

0g FV

Chicken chop (bone-in)- 7 oz

cauliflower florets- ½_cup

mixed greens- 1 cup

Sherry Vinaigrette- 2 Tbsp

4.6g Net Carbs

4.2g FV

Conclusion:

The human civilization has come across a number of alterations, changes, and transitions. These alterations have moved the whole mankind towards an ever growing era of progress. Every item of survival is now backed by survival. But even today the need for nourishment stands as the basic and most innate need of mankind. This basic need had been a part of human nature since the birth of very first man on this planet. Modern man though progressing at a rapid speed cannot deny from this preliminary need of survival.

number of various new modes of nourishment. Today the dietary industry has proliferated into a large domain where hundreds of products are available for nourishing and full filling the basic need. These products ensure quick and easy solutions for eating. But the extensive use of these processed items has moved this generation towards obesity and extensive rate of weight gain. Even the youngest segment of the population is also reporting obesity and extra pounds over the body. It is because our eating habits have been ruined by this pattern of living where everything is mechanized. Atkins diet is like a ray of hope for all those who have lost their hearts against weight loss struggle. The majority of the diet plans make a person victim of starvation hence progress is very disheartening. Atkins diet is the eventual cure for all kind of weight loss issues along with the attainment of healthy lifestyle.

Don't forget to grab our free weight loss report to maximize your chances of success at
flatbellyqueens.com

You may also like these books...

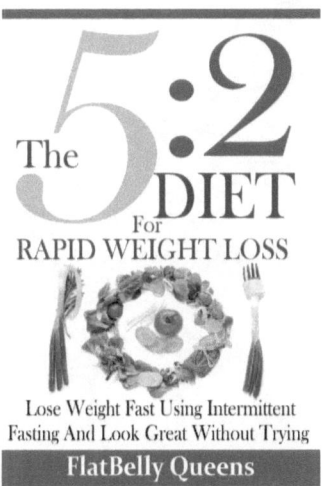

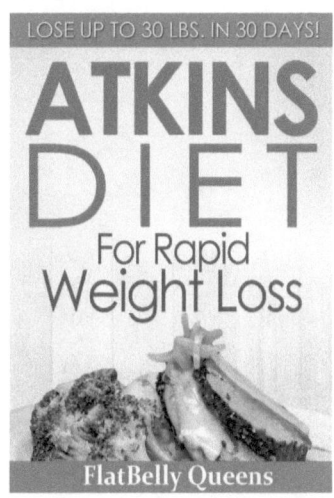

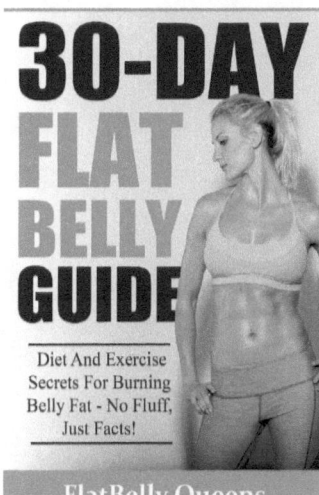

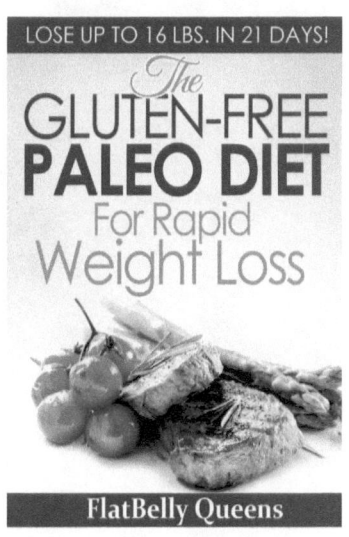